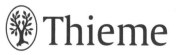

# Neurosurgery Outlines

**Paul E. Kaloostian, MD, FAANS, FACS**
Assistant Professor of Neurosurgery
University of California, Riverside
School of Medicine
Riverside, California, USA

**Christ Ordookhanian, BS**
MD Candidate
University of California, Riverside
School of Medicine
Riverside, California, USA

349 illustrations

Thieme
New York • Stuttgart • Delhi • Rio de Janeiro

**Library of Congress Cataloging-in-Publication Data** is available with the publisher.

Thieme Publishers New York
333 Seventh Avenue, New York, NY 10001 USA
+1 800 782 3488, customerservice@thieme.com

Georg Thieme Verlag KG
Rüdigerstrasse 14, 70469 Stuttgart, Germany
+49 [0]711 8931 421, customerservice@thieme.de

Thieme Publishers Delhi
A-12, Second Floor, Sector-2, Noida-201301
Uttar Pradesh, India
+91 120 45 566 00, customerservice@thieme.in

Thieme Publishers Rio de Janeiro,
Thieme Publicações Ltda.
Edifício Rodolpho de Paoli, 25° andar
Av. Nilo Peçanha, 50 – Sala 2508,
Rio de Janeiro 20020-906 Brasil
+55 21 3172-2297

Cover design: Thieme Publishing Group
Typesetting by DiTech Process Solutions, India

Printed in USA by King Printing Company, Inc.
5 4 3 2 1

ISBN 978-1-68420-142-6

Also available as an e-book:
eISBN 978-1-68420-143-3

**Important note:** Medicine is an ever-changing science undergoing continual development. Research and clinical experience are continually expanding our knowledge, in particular our knowledge of proper treatment and drug therapy. Insofar as this book mentions any dosage or application, readers may rest assured that the authors, editors, and publishers have made every effort to ensure that such references are in accordance with **the state of knowledge at the time of production of the book.**

Nevertheless, this does not involve, imply, or express any guarantee or responsibility on the part of the publishers in respect to any dosage instructions and forms of applications stated in the book. **Every user is requested to examine carefully** the manufacturers' leaflets accompanying each drug and to check, if necessary in consultation with a physician or specialist, whether the dosage schedules mentioned therein or the contraindications stated by the manufacturers differ from the statements made in the present book. Such examination is particularly important with drugs that are either rarely used or have been newly released on the market. Every dosage schedule or every form of application used is entirely at the user's own risk and responsibility. The authors and publishers request every user to report to the publishers any discrepancies or inaccuracies noticed. If errors in this work are found after publication, errata will be posted at www.thieme.com on the product description page.

Some of the product names, patents, and registered designs referred to in this book are in fact registered trademarks or proprietary names even though specific reference to this fact is not always made in the text. Therefore, the appearance of a name without designation as proprietary is not to be construed as a representation by the publisher that it is in the public domain.

FSC
www.fsc.org
100%
Paper from well-managed forests
FSC® C103101

*To our patients, thank you for the distinct opportunity to be a part of your lives and for the privilege to walk alongside you throughout your treatment. Your contribution to our development and medical literature is a priceless entity we share. To our families and friends, we thank you for your endless support and wisdom.*

# Contents

# Contents

## Section III: Cranial Lesion Resection (Brain Tumor, Vascular Lesions)

# Contents

## Section V: Functional Neurosurgery

## Section VI: Epilepsy

# Contents

## Section VII: Pain Management Strategies

## Section VIII: Hydrocephalus Treatment

# Contents

# Contributors

**Ryan F. Amidon, BS**
Junior Specialist (Dr. Garret Anderson Laboratory)
Department of Neuroscience
University of California
Riverside, California, USA

**Paul E. Kaloostian, MD, FAANS, FACS**
Assistant Professor of Neurosurgery
University of California, Riverside
School of Medicine
Riverside, California, USA

**Christ Ordookhanian, BS**
MD Candidate
University of California, Riverside
School of Medicine
Riverside, California, USA

# Section I

## Spine

# 1 Cervical

*Christ Ordookhanian and Paul E. Kaloostian*

## 1.1 Trauma

### 1.1.1 Anterior Cervical Fusion/Posterior Cervical Fusion

#### Indications

- Traumatic occipitoatlantal disjointment
- No complete arch of C1
- Bursting C1 fracture (see ▶ Fig. 1.1)
- Congenital abnormalities
- Odontoid movement into foramen magnum
- Vertebral shifts

#### Symptoms and Signs

- Stiff neck
- Sharp pinpoint pain in neck
- Soreness lasting >7 days
- Weakness in neck muscle
- Tingling/Numbness in general neck area
- Trouble gripping objects
- Tingling in finger tips
- Frequent tension headaches (~4+ days per week)

#### Surgical Pathology

- Traumatic brain injury (TBI)
- Traumatic injury to general neck region
  - Fracture/Displacement/Compression

#### Surgical Procedure

1. Informed consent signed, preoperative labs normal, no Aspirin/Plavix/ Coumadin/other anticoagulants for at least 12 days
2. Appropriate intubation and sedation
3. Horizontal skin incision 1 to 2 inches on either side of the spine
4. Split thin muscle underlying skin

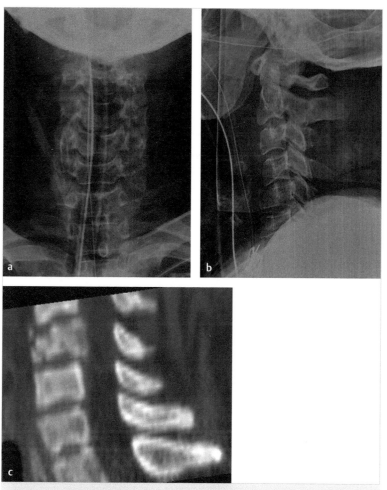

**Fig. 1.1** **(a–c)** A man suffered an incomplete cord injury after a vehicle crash. Radiology revealed that his cervical trauma was a C5 complete burst fracture. (Source: Diagnostic Features. In: Vialle L, ed. AOSpine Masters Series, Volume 5: Cervical Spine Trauma. 1st ed. Thieme; 2015).

5. Enter plane between sternocleidomastoid muscle and strap muscle
6. (Anterior) Enter into the plane between trachea/esophagus and carotid sheath
7. Dissect away thin fascia

8. Locate disk (preoperative imaging match/intraoperative fluoroscopy)
9. Remove disk by cutting annulus fibrosis and nucleus pulposus
10. Remove entire disk including cartilage endplates to reveal cortical bone
11. Remove ligamentous tissue front to back to allow access to spinal canal
12. Insert bone graft and implant cage into evacuated space
13. Attach small plate to front of spine with screws in each vertebral bone (see ▸ Fig. 1.2 to ▸ Fig. 1.4)
14. Clean surgical site, exit, and suture
15. If posterior approach is needed, place the patient prone with Mayfield head pins with all pressure points padded
16. Dissect to lamina over affected levels and confirm levels on X-ray
17. Perform laminectomy and foraminotomies over affected levels that are stenotic and place lateral mass screws with rods and bone graft if needed over affected levels for fusion
18. Obtain hemostasis, place drain, and close wound in multiple layers

## Pitfalls

- Loss of neck mobility by ~30%
- Intraoperative cerebrospinal fluid (CSF) leak

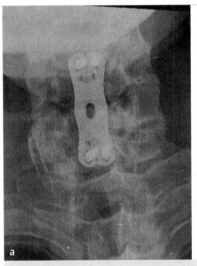 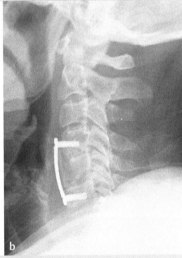

**Fig. 1.2** (a, b) Cord decompression, corpectomy (C5), and fusion (C4–C6) were performed. The fusion healed within one year. (Source: Diagnostic Features. In: Vialle L, ed. AOSpine Masters Series, Volume 5: Cervical Spine Trauma. 1st ed. Thieme; 2015).

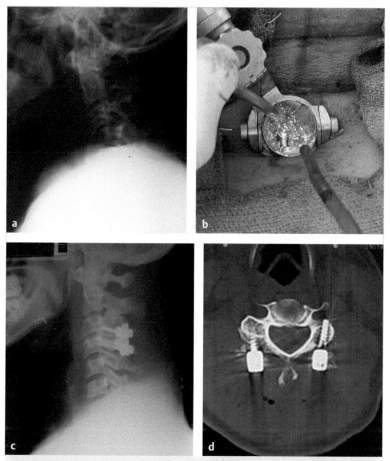

**Fig. 1.3** (a–d) A patient suffered cervical trauma resulting in C3/C4 dislocation. Fusion (C3–C4) was performed and lateral mass screw placement was verified using X-ray and CT scan. (Source: Cervical case studies. In: Perez-Cruet M, Fessler R, Wang M, eds. An Anatomic Approach to Minimally Invasive Spine Surgery. 2nd ed. Thieme; 2018).

- Blood clot (deep vein thrombosis, or more severe pulmonary embolism)
- Damage to spinal nerves and/or cord
- Postoperative weakness or numbness or continued pain
- Postoperative wound infection
- Continued symptoms postsurgically/unresolved symptoms with no improvement to quality of life

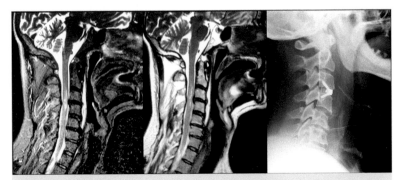

**Fig. 1.4** A man suffered cervical trauma after a bicycle accident, resulting in traumatic disk herniation. Radiology revealed associated cord contusion and C3–C4 instability. Fusion (C3–C4) was performed and after therapy, his paresis reduced. (Source: Brembilla C, Lanterna L, Gritti P, et al. The use of a stand-alone interbody fusion cage in subaxial cervical spine trauma: a preliminary report. J Neurol Surg A Cent Eur Neurosurg 2015;76(01):13–19).

## Prognosis

- Most patient are hospitalized for 1 to 2 days, then return home with strict orders of minimal sudden head/neck movement
- Typically, 4 to 6 weeks post operation most patients are able to return to normal day-to-day activities
- Full fusion (formation of hard bone) may take 12 to 18 months
- Physical therapy (PT) and occupational therapy (OT) should strongly be considered

# 1.2 Elective

## 1.2.1 Anterior Cervical Fusion/Posterior Cervical Fusion

### Indications

- No complete arch of C1
- Bursting C1 fracture
- Congenital abnormalities
- Odontoid movement into foramen magnum
- Vertebral shifts

## Symptoms and Signs

- Stiff neck
- Sharp pinpoint pain in neck
- Soreness lasting >7 days
- Weakness in neck muscle
- Tingling/Numbness in general neck area
- Trouble gripping objects
- Tingling in finger tips
- Frequent tension headaches (~4+ days per week)

## Surgical Pathology

- Spondylosis
- Spondylosis
- Adjacent segment pathology (ASP)
- Radiculopathy (see ▶ Fig. 1.5)
- Osteomyelitis
- Vertebral body tumors
- Myelopathy (see ▶ Fig. 1.6 and ▶ Fig. 1.7)
- Postlaminectomy kyphosis (see ▶ Fig. 1.8)
- Opacified posterior longitudinal ligament

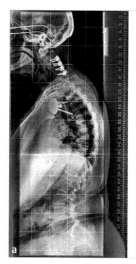
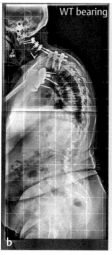

Fig. 1.5 (a, b) An elderly woman with neck pain and deformity from myelopathy received posterior decompression (C3–C6), anterior diskectomy and fusion (C4–C5), and posterior fusion (C2–T2). A transition rod was added for stabilization. (Source: Radiographic considerations. In: Ames C, Riew K, Abumi K, eds. Cervical Spine Deformity Surgery. 1st ed. Thieme; 2019).

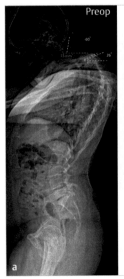 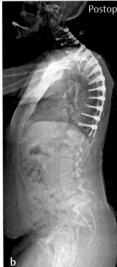

**Fig. 1.6** (a, b) An elderly man with chin-on-chest deformity (kyphosis) received anterior and posterior cervical osteotomies. Posterior fusion (C2–T10) was performed and resulted in significant correction of the kyphosis. (Source: Radiographic considerations. In: Ames C, Riew K, Abumi K, eds. Cervical Spine Deformity Surgery. 1st ed. Thieme; 2019).

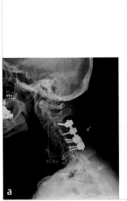 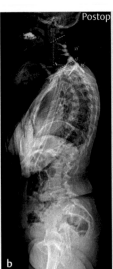

**Fig. 1.7** (a, b) An elderly woman with neck pain from myelopathy received posterior decompression and fusion (C3–C6). This was followed by a diskectomy and osteotomy (C6–C7), posterior fusion (C2–T2), and laminectomy (C6/7 and C7/T1) for decompression. (Source: Radiographic considerations. In: Ames C, Riew K, Abumi K, eds. Cervical Spine Deformity Surgery. 1st ed. Thieme; 2019).

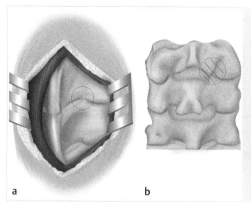

**Fig. 1.8** (a, b) Landmarks for posterior cervical tubular decompression via foraminotomy. After identifying the lamina–facet junction and other bony landmarks, commence laminar resection. (Source: Minimally invasive tubular posterior cervical decompressive techniques. In: Vaccaro A, Albert T, eds. Spine Surgery: Tricks of the Trade. 3rd ed. Thieme; 2016).

a                          b

## Surgical Procedure

1. Informed consent signed, preoperative labs normal, no Aspirin/Plavix/Coumadin/other anticoagulants for at least 12 days
2. Appropriate intubation and sedation
3. Horizontal skin incision 1 to 2 inches on either side of spine
4. Split thin muscle underlying skin
5. Enter the plane between sternocleidomastoid muscle and strap muscle
6. (Anterior) Enter into the plane between trachea/esophagus and carotid sheath
7. Disect away thin fascia
8. Locate disk (preoperative imaging match/intraoperative fluoroscopy)
9. Remove disk by cutting annulus fibrosis and nucleus pulposus
10. Remove entire disk including cartilage endplates to reveal cortical bone
11. Remove ligamentous tissue front to back to allow access to spinal canal
12. (Posterior) Incision on midline, behind neck
13. Elevate paraspinal muscles
14. Confirm correct level (discussed above)
15. Remove small portion of facet joint with burr drill, expose nerve root, gently move to side to expose disk herniation
16. Insert bone graft and implant cage into evacuated space
17. Attach small plate to spine with screws in each vertebral bone
18. Clean surgical site, exit, and suture

## Pitfalls

- Loss of neck mobility by ~30%
- Instrumentation failure
- Bone graft failure
- Intraoperative CSF leak
- Blood clot (deep vein thrombosis, or more severe pulmonary embolism)
- Damage to spinal nerves and/or cord
- Postoperative weakness or numbness or continued pain
- Postoperative wound infection
- Continued symptoms postsurgically/unresolved symptoms with no improvement to quality of life

## Prognosis

- Most patient are hospitalized for 1 to 2 days, then return home with strict orders of minimal sudden head/neck movement
- Typically, 4 to 6 weeks post operation most patients are able to return to normal day-to-day activities
- Full fusion (formation of hard bone) may take 12 to 18 months
- PT and OT

# 1.2.2 Posterior Cervical Foraminotomy/Posterior Cervical Decompression

## Symptoms and Signs

- Mild to moderate neck pain
- Radicular sensory loss in arm(s)
- Radicular pain in arm(s)
- Myotomal weakness in arm(s)
- Myelopathy (dropping objects, cannot button shirt, gait imbalance, and urinary incontinence)

## Surgical Pathology

- Cervical herniated nucleus pulposus
- Foraminal stenosis
- Cord compression

## Diagnostic Modalities

- X-ray of cervical spine to assess for alignment, fracture, and degenerative disease

- CT of cervical spine to assess for bony anatomy regarding alignment, fracture, and degenerative disease
- MRI of cervical spine to assess for nerve root or cord compression
- Dynamic X-ray of cervical spine to look for instability (in patients without severe cord compression)

## Differential Diagnosis

- Degenerative disease
- Traumatic nerve root compression

## Treatment Options

- Exhaust all conservative routes with PT, aqua therapy, chiropractic, acupuncture, epidural steroid injections, and medical management (if possible, prior to surgical intervention)
- Surgical decompression with or without stabilization via posterior decompression and foraminotomy (at appropriate indicated levels based on imaging studies)

## Indications for Surgical Intervention

- Intractable radicular arm pain
- Intractable weakness and/or numbness in arms in radicular fashion
- Cord compression with or without myelopathy

## Surgical Procedure for Posterior Cervical Spine

1. Informed consent signed, preoperative labs normal, no Aspirin/Plavix/Coumadin/other anticoagulants for at least 2 weeks preoperatively
2. Appropriate intubation and sedation
3. Place the patient prone in neutral position with Mayfield head holder
4. Time out performed
5. Incision along posterior cervical spine midline
6. Subperiosteal dissection of muscles down to bone performed at appropriate level (see ▶ Fig. 1.9)
7. X-ray/fluoroscopic confirmation with two people for appropriate level (see ▶ Fig. 1.10)
8. Laminectomy and foraminotomy unilaterally or bilaterally, if needed, depending on diagnosis and indication for surgery (see ▶ Fig. 1.11)
   a. Use pituitary rongeur/Kerrison rongeur and high-speed drill

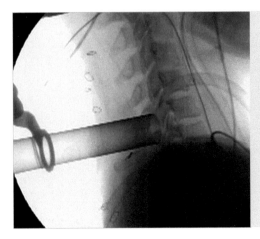

**Fig. 1.9** Fluoroscopy reveals trajectory of tube for cervical decompression. Identify the facet joint before placing parallel to disk space at that level. (Source: Minimally invasive tubular posterior cervical decompressive techniques. In: Vaccaro A, Albert T, eds. Spine Surgery: Tricks of the Trade. 3rd ed. Thieme; 2016).

9. Once spinal cord and/or nerve roots are decompressed, obtain X-ray confirming appropriate levels decompressed
10. If stabilization is planned, then instrumentation and fusion can be performed
11. Muscle and skin closure with drain placed (if necessary)

## Pitfalls

- Intraoperative CSF leak
- Blood clot (deep vein thrombosis, or more severe pulmonary embolism)
- Damage to spinal nerves and/or cord
- Postoperative weakness or numbness or continued pain
- Postoperative wound infection
- Continued symptoms postsurgically/unresolved symptoms with no improvement to quality of life

## Prognosis

- Most patient are discharged home the same day for single level foraminotomy
- Typically, 4 to 6 weeks post operation most patients are able to return to normal day-to-day activities
- PT/OT can be performed as outpatient to regain strength
- Most patients do very well and are happy with the results

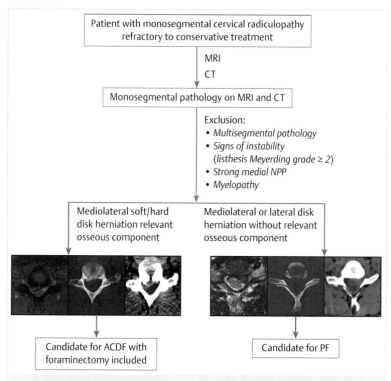

**Fig. 1.10** Guide for patient selection considering between anterior cervical diskectomy and fusion (ACDF) and posterior foraminotomy (PF). Patients selected for PF will have mediolateral or lateral disk herniation and are without relevant osseous component. (Source: Scholz T, Geiger M, Mainz V, et al. Anterior cervical decompression and fusion or posterior foraminotomy for cervical radiculopathy: results of a single-center series. J Neurol Surg A Cent Eur Neurosurg 2018;79(03):211–217).

# 1.3 Tumor/Vascular

## 1.3.1 Cervical Tumor Resection (Vertebral Pathology)

### Symptoms and Signs

- Incidental with symptoms (depending on size and location)
- Moderate/Severe numbness in upper extremities

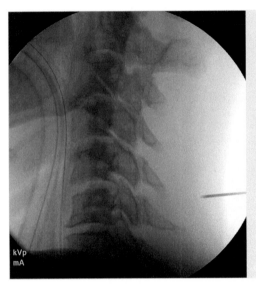

**Fig. 1.11** A spinal needle marks entrance site for a lower cervical (C6–C7) foraminotomy. It is recommended to enter the skin rostral to the foramen. (Source: Operative procedure. In: Wolfla C, Resnick D, eds. Neurosurgical Operative Atlas: Spine and Peripheral Nerves. 3rd ed. Thieme; 2016).

- Paresthesias in upper body extremities
- Neck pain and loss of mobility due to neck pain
- Radiating pain down the arms
- Pain in moving shoulders
- Muscle weakness in arms
- Inability to conduct fine motor skills with hands

## Surgical Pathology

- Cervical spine benign/malignant tumor

## Diagnostic Modalities

- CT of cervical spine with and without contrast to assess whether there is bony involvement of tumor
- MRI of cervical spine with and without contrast to assess if there is spinal cord, epidural space, or nerve root involvement of tumor
- PET scan of body to look for other foci of tumor
- CT of chest/abdomen/pelvis to rule out metastatic disease

## Differential Diagnosis

- Metastatic tumor
  - Breast, prostate, lung, renal cell

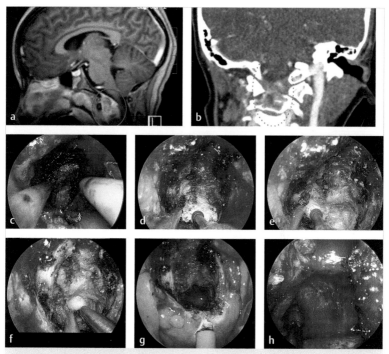

**Fig. 1.12** (**a–h**) Higher cervical (C2) resection of giant cell tumor via endoscopic transnasal and transoral approaches. Radiology reveals the location of the tumor. Gross total tumor resection was achieved. (Source: Surgical technique. In: Stamm A, ed. Transnasal Endoscopic Skull Base and Brain Surgery: Surgical Anatomy and Its Applications. 2nd ed. Thieme; 2019).

- Primary tumor (see ▶ Fig. 1.12)
  - Schwannoma, myeloma, plasmacytoma, meningioma

## Treatment Options

- Acute pain control with medications and pain management
- If asymptomatic or mildly symptomatic with neck pain/radiculopathy with small focus of tumor:
  - Radiation treatment (radiation oncology consultation)
  - Chemotherapy (medical oncology consultation)
  - Kyphoplasty (to treat pain)

- Surgical instrumentation and fusion (if there is concern for deformity, instability, or cord compression)
- If symptomatic with cord compression and myelopathy with large tumor burden:
  - Urgent surgical decompression and fusion over multiple segments with tumor resection if deemed suitable candidate for surgery; may be followed by radiation treatment after resection if considered necessary by the radiation oncologist
    - The oncologist will need to determine overall prognosis, Karnofsky performance score, and extent of visceral disease
    - If poor surgical candidate with poor life expectancy, medical management is recommended
    - Surgery may be done anteriorly, posteriorly, or combined two-stage approach for added stabilization (see ▶ Fig. 1.13)
  - Preoperative embolization may be indicated for select vascular tumors to the spine such as renal cell cancer, thyroid cancer, breast cancer, etc. in order to decrease vascularity intraoperatively

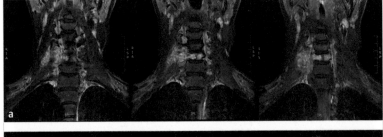
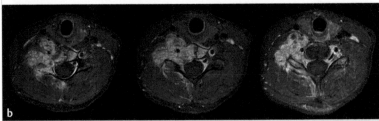

**Fig. 1.13** (a, b) Radiology revealed presence of lower cervical tumor in teenage girl who presented with symptoms of myelopathy. Tumor embolization, anterior corpectomy (C6) with tumor resection and reconstruction, and fusion (C4–C6) were performed. Improved alignment was achieved and the tumor was confirmed to be totally resected. (Source: Introduction and background. In: Cohen A, ed. Pediatric Neurosurgery: Tricks of the Trade. 1st ed. Thieme; 2015).

## Indications for Surgical Intervention

- Intractable neck and radicular pain refractory to all conservative routes
- Cord compression with or without myelopathy
- To obtain diagnosis if no other site for biopsy is available

## Surgical Procedure for Posterior Cervical Spine

1. Informed consent signed, preoperative labs normal, no Aspirin/Plavix/Coumadin/other anticoagulants for at least 2 weeks for elective cases
2. Appropriate intubation and sedation and lines (if necessary) as per the anesthetist
3. Patient placed prone with Mayfield pins in neutral alignment on Jackson Table with all pressure points padded
4. Neuromonitoring may be present to monitor nerves (if necessary and indicated)
5. Time out is performed with agreement from everyone in the room for correct patient and correct surgery with consent signed
6. Make an incision over the vertebrae where laminectomy is to be performed
7. Perform subperiosteal dissection of muscles bilaterally to expose the vertebra
8. Once the bone is exposed, it is best to localize and verify the correct vertebra via X-ray or fluoroscopic imaging and confirming with at least two people in the room
9. Perform the laminectomy over segments needed based on preoperative imaging of levels that are compressed due to tumor:
   a. Using Leksell rongeurs and hand-held high-speed drill, remove the bony spinous process and bilateral lamina as indicated for specific procedure
   b. Remove the thick ligamentum flavum with Kerrison rongeurs with careful dissection beneath the ligament to ensure no adhesions exist to dura mater below and thus avoiding CSF leak
   c. Perform appropriate foraminotomy with Kerosen rongeurs as needed for appropriate decompression of nerve roots
   d. Identify location of tumor and resect tumor as needed if within the lamina, epidural, or within the spinal canal/cord:
      i. If within the lamina or epidural in nature, the tumor can be visualized immediately and removed gently
      ii. If within the spinal cord, use operative microscope and open the spinal cord dura midline with 11 blade and tack up the dural leaflets with suture

iii. If tumor is intradural and extramedullary, it can be resected carefully with microdissection technique without cord injury (neuromonitoring needed in these cases) (see ▶ Fig. 1.14)

iv. If tumor is intradural and intramedullary, with microdissection technique the cord must be entered midline and the tumor must be identified and resected starting centrally first, then around the edges (neuromonitoring needed in these cases)

10. After appropriate tumor resection, there may be need for additional stabilization to prevent kyphosis if the resection caused multiple segment decompression. Therefore, instrumentation with lateral mass screws can be placed over the segments involved with rods bilaterally and fusion/arthrodesis along these segments. (see ▶ Fig. 1.15 and ▶ Fig. 1.16)

11. After appropriate hemostasis is obtained, muscle and skin incisions can then be closed in appropriate fashion, often with placement of postoperative drains that can be removed after 2 to 3 days.

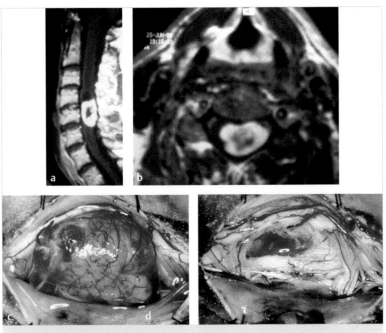

**Fig. 1.14 (a–d)** Radiology revealed tumor at the C5 level, accompanying severe cord compression. After dissecting to the tumor, it was successfully resected. (Source: Intradural extramedullary tumors. In: Bernstein M, Berger M, eds. Neuro-oncology: The Essentials. 3rd ed. Thieme; 2014).

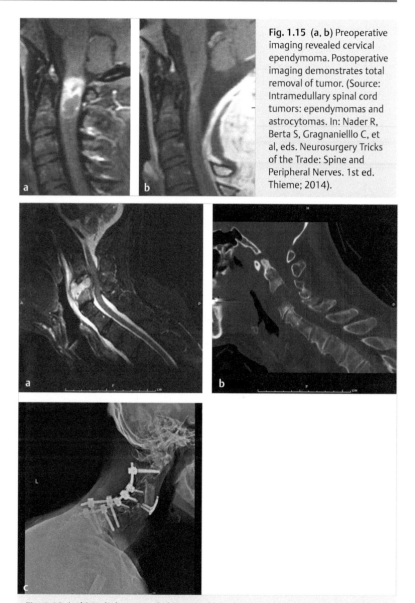

**Fig. 1.15 (a, b)** Preoperative imaging revealed cervical ependymoma. Postoperative imaging demonstrates total removal of tumor. (Source: Intramedullary spinal cord tumors: ependymomas and astrocytomas. In: Nader R, Berta S, Gragnaniello C, et al, eds. Neurosurgery Tricks of the Trade: Spine and Peripheral Nerves. 1st ed. Thieme; 2014).

**Fig. 1.16 (a, b)** Radiology revealed a cervical lymphoma and lysis of C3 in an elderly man. Anterior corpectomy and posterior stabilization were performed and confirmed via postoperative CT scan. (Source: Vertebral bone tumors. In: Fessler R, Sekhar L, eds. Atlas of Neurosurgical Techniques: Spine and Peripheral Nerves. 2nd ed. Thieme; 2016).

## Pitfalls

- Loss of neck mobility (minimal, unless fusion extended to occiput and C1)
- Intraoperative CSF leak
- Blood clot (deep vein thrombosis, or more severe pulmonary embolism)
- Damage to spinal nerves and/or cord
- Postoperative weakness or numbness or continued pain
- Postoperative wound infection
- Continued symptoms postsurgically/unresolved symptoms with no improvement to quality of life
- Prolonged hospitalization due to invasiveness of surgery and other comorbidities/iatrogenic infection

## Prognosis

- Hospitalization rates depend on the type of procedure performed, preoperative examination status, and patient's age/comorbidities
- PT and OT will be needed postoperatively, immediately and as outpatient to regain strength
- Brace/collar is used for 8 weeks after discharge to immobilize to increase rate of healing

## 1.3.2 Cervical Vascular Lesion Treatment for Arteriovenous Malformation (AVM) (Vertebral Pathology)

### Symptoms and Signs (AVM)

- Dilated arteries and veins with dysplastic vessels
- Subarachnoid hemorrhage
- Neck pain and loss of mobility due to neck pain
- Pain in moving shoulders
- Meningism (neck rigidity, photophobia, and headache)
- Myelopathy
- Seizure
- Ischemic injury to cervical
- Increased sweating around cervical vascular lesion
- Hemorrhaging
- Inability to conduct fine motor skills with hands

## Surgical Pathology

- Cervical vascular benign/malignant lesions

## Diagnostic Modalities

- Angiography:
  - Preoperative spinal angiography
  - Intraoperative indocyanine green (ICG) angiography
- CT of cervical spine with and without contrast (can rule out acute hemorrhage)
- MRI of cervical spine with and without contrast

## Differential Diagnosis:

- Fibromuscular dysplasia (FMD):
  - Craniocervical FMD
- Spinal AVM (see ▶ Fig. 1.17 and ▶ Fig. 1.18):
  - Intradural-intramedullary (hemorrhaging common)
    ○ Glomus (Type II) (see ▶ Fig. 1.19 and ▶ Fig. 1.20)
    ○ Juvenile (Type III)
  - Intradural-extramedullary
  - Conus medullaris
  - Metameric
  - Extradural
  - Cavernoma
  - Capillary telangiectasia
- Spinal dural arteriovenous fistula (AVF, Type I) (see ▶ Fig. 1.21):
  - Intradural-extramedullary
    ○ Perimedullary AVF (Type IV)
  - Intradural-intramedullary
  - Extradural
- Vertebral sarcoidosis
- Dissection syndromes:
  - Cervical internal carotid artery
  - Extracranial vertebral artery

## Treatment Options

- Conservative observation
- Radiation treatment:
  - Conventional radiation: not very effective therapy

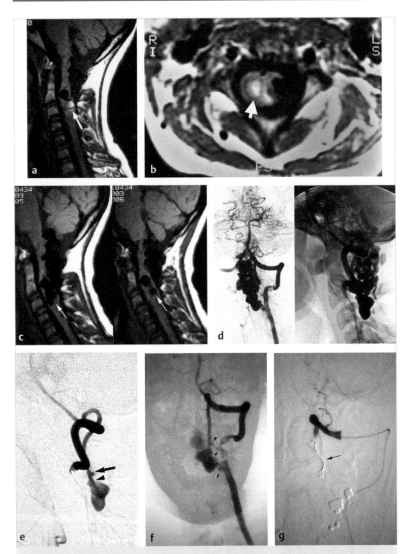

**Fig. 1.17 (a–g)** Radiology revealed an upper cervical intradural arteriovenous fistula (AVF) with an aneurysm in a teenage girl. Several feeding vessels were identified at the fistula. The fistula was surgically treated after reducing its blood flow by placing a coil in the main feeding artery. (Source: Operative procedure. In: Macdonald R, ed. Neurosurgical Operative Atlas: Vascular Neurosurgery. 3rd ed. Thieme; 2018).

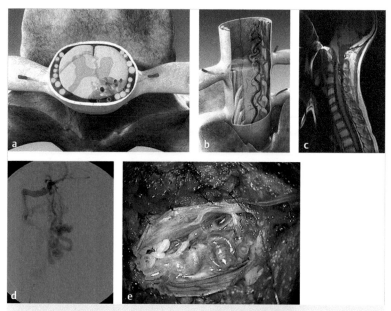

**Fig. 1.18 (a–e)** Radiology revealed a cervical diffuse intramedullary arteriovenous malformation (AVM) in a teenage boy. Feeding vessels were identified to be from the anterior spinal artery and muscular branches. (Source: Relevant anatomy and classification. In: Spetzler R, Kalani M, Nakaji P, eds. Neurovascular Surgery. 2nd ed. Thieme; 2015).

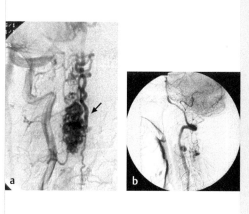

**Fig. 1.19 (a, b)** Preoperative angiography revealed an unresectable type 2 cervical arteriovenous malformation (AVM). Postoperative angiography (24 months) demonstrates successful treatment of nidus via stereotactic radiosurgery. (Source: Stereotactic radiosurgery of spinal arteriovenous malformations. In: Nader R, Berta S, Gragnaniellllo C, et al, eds. Neurosurgery Tricks of the Trade: Spine and Peripheral Nerves. 1st ed. Thieme; 2014).

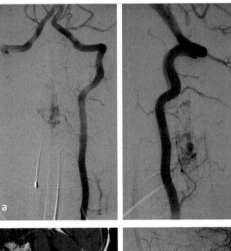
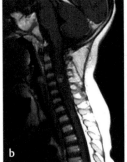
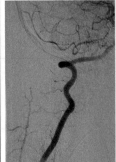

**Fig. 1.20** (a, b) Preoperative angiography and magnetic resonance imaging (MRI) revealed cervical intramedullary arteriovenous malformation (AVM), commonly referred to as glomus AVMs. Postoperative angiography demonstrates successful treatment of AVM. (Source: Spinal intramedullary arteriovenous malformations. In: Albright A, Pollack I, Adelson P, eds. Principles and Practice of Pediatric Neurosurgery. 3rd ed. Thieme; 2014).

- – Stereotactic radiosurgery and radiotherapy (nidus must not be greater than 3 cm in diameter)
- Surgery:
  - – Microsurgical resection
  - – Preferred option if bleeding or seizures result from lesion
- Endovascular embolization using the following embolic agents (initial procedure to facilitate surgery):
  - – Coils: close down vessel supplying AVM (cannot independently treat AVM nidus)
  - – Onyx: solidifies, forming a cast, in vessel supplying AVM (best penetration of AVM nidus)
  - – NBCA: solidifies as a glue in vessel supplying AVM (greater risks and worse outcomes than with Onyx)

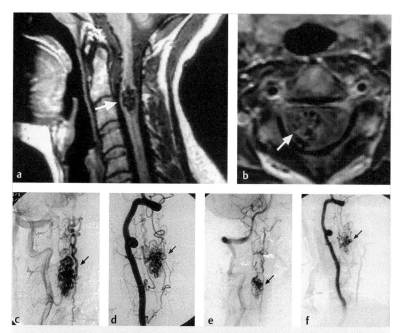

**Fig. 1.21 (a–f)** Magnetic resonance imaging (MRI) revealed an arteriovenous malformation (AVM) at C2–C3 in a middle-aged woman. Cyberknife treatment was performed, reducing the AVM's total volume by 75%. Residual AVM was treated with radiation (15 Gy in two fractions). (Source: Conclusion. In: Dickman C, Fehlings M, Gokaslan Z, eds. Spinal Cord and Spinal Column Tumors. 1st ed. Thieme; 2006).

- – PVA: used prior to craniotomy or surgical resection of AVM (cannot independently treat AVM pathology)
- Combination techniques:
  - – Embolization followed by stereotactic radiosurgery
- Venous angiomas should not be treated unless certainly contributing to intractable seizures and bleeding

## Indications for Endovascular Intervention

- Preoperative embolization (for surgical AVM resection)
- Presence of associated lesions (aneurysms/pseudoaneurysms on feeding pedicle or nidus, venous thrombosis, venous outflow restriction, venous pouches, dilatations)

- Small surgically inaccessible AVM treated by curative AVM embolization or radiosurgery
- Palliative treatment when symptomatic AVM not entirely treatable by the other approaches

## Surgical Procedure for Cervical Spine (Laminoplasty)

1. Administer propranolol 20 mg orally four times a day for 3 days to patient preoperation
2. Informed consent signed, preoperative labs normal, no Aspirin/Plavix/ Coumadin/NSAIDs/Celebrex/Naprosyn/other anticoagulants and anti-inflammatory drugs for at least 2 weeks
3. Administer preoperative prophylactic intravenous (IV) antibiotics
4. Appropriate intubation and sedation and lines (if necessary, as per the anesthetist)
5. Patient placed prone on gel rolls, with head clamped via Mayfield pins, pressure points padded, and any hair clipped over upper cervical region
6. Neuromonitoring may be required to monitor nerves (if necessary and indicated)
7. Eyes taped closed and Bair Hugger covers upper body
8. Time out is performed with agreement from everyone in the room for correct patient and correct surgery with consent signed
9. C-arm fluoroscopy equipment set up in operation zone
10. Make an incision over the vertebrae where laminoplasty is to be performed:
    a. Prepare to utilize one level above and below the AVM nidus or AVF shunt
    b. Extension to ipsilateral pedicle performed if deemed necessary to enhance lateral of the AVM nidus or AVF shunt
11. Perform subperiosteal dissection of muscles bilaterally to expose the vertebra
12. Once the bone is exposed, it is best to localize and verify the correct vertebra via X-ray or fluoroscopic imaging and confirming with at least two people in the room
13. Bovie electrocautery is used to progress dissection toward the spine and to attain hemostasis, with the help of bipolar forceps
14. Move musculature around vertebra laterally and downward to expose the dura
15. Utilize self-retaining retractors to keep everything in place
16. Open the dura, followed by the arachnoid
17. Clip the arachnoid to the dural edges using self-retaining retractors to reveal the AVM

18. Video-angiography (typically with ICG) is used to visualize the blood flow through the AVM
19. If the AVM nidus is intraparenchymal in its entirety, prepare to perform a myelotomy (midline dorsal, dorsal root entry zone, lateral, and anterior midline types). Otherwise, continue with the laminoplasty procedure (typically a pial resection).
20. Using the surgical suction and nonstick bipolar forceps, the pia arachnoid is revealed
21. Cut and coagulate the appropriate vessels
22. Separate AVM from the spinal cord using surgical scissors, bipolar, and suction
23. Several nerve rootlets will be tangled with the AVM (they may be tangled with dorsal nerve roots) and must be removed by necessity; others may be left unaltered
24. Cut the dentate ligament where it is attached to the AVM
25. The spinal canal is further exposed, revealing the feeders of the AVM
26. Use video-angiography to confirm no further shunting of the arterial venous blood
27. Close the dura as well as the subcutaneous tissues after the laminoplasty is successfully performed
28. Close the skin with suture, skin-glue, steri-strips, or surgical staples
29. Postoperative injection of the vertebral artery and the thyrocervical trunk demonstrate that the AVM has been treated

## Surgical Procedure for Cervical Spine (Laminectomy)

1. Follow AVM laminoplasty procedure above until initial hemostasis is completed and self-retaining retractors are placed, keeping the musculature set aside
2. Use Leksell rongeurs and high-speed burr drill to remove the posterior spinous processes and bilateral lamina
3. Remove the free ligamentum flavum using Kerrison rongeurs to decompress the nerve roots
4. Open the lamina via "green-stick" fracture technique
5. Utilizing Adson Periosteal Elevator, elevate lamina from the side (do not slide underneath it)
6. Fasten plates and screws at the lateral borders of each lamina and the facet joint, decompressing the spinal cord (if needed, often fusion is not necessary)
7. Wash out the wound with antibiotic saline solution and reachieve hemostasis via Bovie electrocautery and bipolar, applying local anesthetic to the wound to reduce bleeding

8. Place a postoperative drain (can be removed after 2–3 days)
9. Close the fascia and subcutaneous tissue with Vicryl
10. Close the skin with suture, skin-glue, steri-strips, or surgical staples

## Embolization Procedure (Onyx)

1. Shake Onyx vial on mixer for 20 minutes. Onyx-18 is common, Onyx-34 is suitable for very high flow AVMs, and Onyx-500 is incorporated in aneurysm embolization treatments
2. Wedge microcatheter tip into arterial branch supplying the AVM, preferably very close to the AVM nidus
3. Perform angiography through the microcatheter to confirm that the arterial branch exclusively supplies the AVM
4. Prime the dimethyl sulfoxide (DMSO)-compatible microcatheter (marathon, echelon, rebar, ultraflow) with 0.3 to 0.8 mL DMSO so that Onyx does not solidify in the microcatheter
5. Slowly inject Onyx solution, allowing no more than 1 cm of reflux. If reflux occurs, continue after a 1 to 2 minutes waiting period
6. Halt injection when Onyx no longer flows into the nidus, but refluxes instead

## Pitfalls

- Stroke
- Intraoperative and postoperative bleeding
- Failure to remove the entire AVM
- Future recurrence of AVM
- Recompression of cervical spinal cord
- Postlaminoplasty kyphosis
- Nerve root palsies
- Damage to spinal nerves and/or cord
- Postoperative weakness or numbness or continued pain
- Postoperative wound infection
- Prolonged hospitalization due to invasiveness of surgery and other comorbidities/iatrogenic infection
- Temporary postoperative paresthesia
- Iatrogenic vertebral artery injury during embolization process

## Prognosis (AVM Laminectomy)

- Hospitalization rates depend on the type of procedure performed, preoperative examination status, and patient's age/comorbidities

- PT and OT will be needed postoperatively, immediately and as outpatient to regain strength
- Brace/Collar is used for 8 weeks after discharge to immobilize to increase rate of healing

## 1.3.3 Cervical Anterior and Posterior Techniques for Tumor Resection (Spinal Canal Pathology)

### Symptoms and Signs

- Incidental with symptoms (depending on size and location)
- Moderate/Severe numbness to pain, cold, and heat in upper extremities
- Paresthesia in upper body extremities
- Neck pain and loss of mobility due to neck pain
- Radiating pain down the arms
- Pain in moving shoulders
- Muscle weakness in arms (potentially paralysis)
- Inability to conduct fine motor skills with hands
- Scoliosis

### Surgical Pathology

- Cervical spine benign/malignant tumor

### Diagnostic Modalities

- CT of cervical spine with and without contrast to assess whether there is bony involvement of tumor
- MRI of cervical spine with and without contrast to assess if there is spinal cord, epidural space, or nerve root involvement of tumor
- PET scan of body to look for other foci of tumor
- CT of chest/abdomen/pelvis to rule out metastatic disease
- X-ray (not as reliable for tumor diagnosis)
- Biopsy to examine tissue sample to determine whether tumor is benign or malignant, and what cancer type resulted in the tumor if malignancy is determined

### Differential Diagnosis

- Metastatic tumor
  - Breast, prostate, lung, renal cell
- Primary tumor

- Schwannoma, neurofibroma, myeloma, plasmacytoma, meningioma, ependymoma, astrocytoma, hemangioblastoma, lipoma, dermoid, epidermoid, teratoma, neuroblastoma, oligodendroglioma, cholesteatoma, subependymoma, osteosarcoma, chondrosarcoma, Ewing's sarcoma, chordoma, lymphoma, osteoid osteoma, aneurysmal bone cyst, eosinophilic granuloma, angiolipoma (see ▶Fig. 1.22 and ▶Fig. 1.23)

## Treatment Options

- Acute pain control with medications and pain management

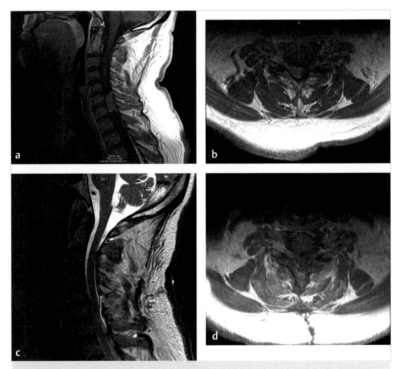

**Fig. 1.22 (a–d)** An elderly man with a dural-based intradural extramedullary tumor (meningioma) received laminoplasty (C6 and C7) and tumor resection treatment. Cord decompression and total tumor resection were achieved. No complications were present at time of discharge. (Source: Spinal meningiomas. In: Sheehan J, Gerszten P, eds. Controversies in Stereotactic Radiosurgery: Best Evidence Recommendations. 1st ed. Thieme; 2014).

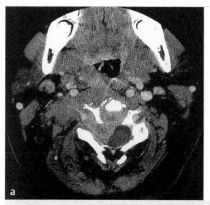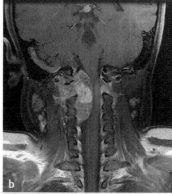

**Fig. 1.23 (a, b)** Computed tomography (CT) scan through C3 revealed cervical extra-dural tumor (chordoma) in a child. Magnetic resonance imaging (MRI) demonstrates cervical cord compression. (Source: Extradural tumors. In: Dickman C, Fehlings M, Gokaslan Z, eds. Spinal Cord and Spinal Column Tumors. 1st ed. Thieme; 2006).

- If asymptomatic or mildly symptomatic with neck pain/radiculopathy with small focus of tumor:
  - Radiation treatment (radiation oncology consultation)
    ○ Some metastatic tumors are radioresistant
  - Chemotherapy (medical oncology consultation)
    ○ Some metastatic tumors are radioresistant
  - Kyphoplasty (to treat pain)
  - Surgical instrumentation and fusion (if there is concern for deformity, instability, or cord compression)
- If symptomatic with cord compression and myelopathy with large tumor burden:
  - Urgent surgical decompression and fusion over multiple segments with tumor resection if deemed suitable candidate for surgery; may be followed by radiation treatment after resection if considered necessary by the radiation oncologist
    ○ The oncologist will need to determine overall prognosis, Karnofsky performance score, and extent of visceral disease
    ○ If poor surgical candidate with poor life expectancy, medical management is recommended
    ○ Surgery may be done anteriorly, posteriorly, or combined two-stage approach for added stabilization
  - Preoperative embolization may be indicated for select vascular tumors to the spine such as renal cell cancer, thyroid cancer, breast cancer, etc. in order to decrease vascularity intraoperatively

## Indications for Surgical Intervention

- Intractable neck and radicular pain refractory to all conservative routes
- Cord compression with or without myelopathy
- To obtain diagnosis if no other site for biopsy is available
- Risk of pathological fractures without stabilization

## Surgical Procedure for Posterior Cervical Spine

1. Informed consent signed, preoperative labs normal, no Aspirin/Plavix/ Coumadin/NSAIDs/Celebrex/Naprosyn/other anticoagulants and anti-inflammatory drugs for at least 2 weeks
2. Appropriate intubation and sedation and lines (if necessary) as per the anesthetist
3. Patient placed prone with Mayfield pins on Jackson Table with all pressure points padded
4. Neuromonitoring is needed
5. Time out is performed with agreement from everyone in the room for correct patient and correct surgery with consent signed
6. Make an incision down the midline of back, over the vertebrae where laminectomy is to be performed
7. Perform subperiosteal dissection of muscles bilaterally to expose the spinous process and paraspinal muscles
8. Dissect tissue planes along spinous process and laminae using rongeurs
9. Move paraspinal muscles laterally to expose the laminae
10. Once the bone is exposed, it is best to localize and verify the correct vertebra via X-ray or fluoroscopic imaging and confirming with at least two people in the room
11. Perform the laminectomy over segments needed based on preoperative imaging of levels that are compressed due to tumor:
    a. Using Leksell rongeurs and hand-held high-speed drill, remove the bony spinous process and bilateral lamina as indicated for specific procedure
    b. Remove the thick ligamentum flavum with Kerrison rongeurs with careful dissection beneath the ligament to ensure no adhesions exist to dura mater below and thus avoiding CSF leak
    c. Perform appropriate foraminotomy with Kerrison rongeurs as needed for appropriate decompression of nerve roots
    d. Identify location of tumor and resect tumor as needed within the spinal canal:
       i. Use operative microscope and open the spinal cord dura midline with 11 blade and tack up the dural leaflets with suture

    ii.  If tumor is intradural and extramedullary, the tumor can then be resected carefully with microdissection technique without cord injury (neuromonitoring needed in these cases)

    iii.  If tumor is intradural and intramedullary, with microdissection technique the cord must be entered midline and the tumor must be identified and resected starting centrally first, then around the edges (neuromonitoring needed in these cases)

12. After appropriate tumor resection, there may be need for additional stabilization to prevent kyphosis if the resection caused multiple segment decompression. Therefore, instrumentation with lateral mass screws can be placed over the segments involved with rods bilaterally and fusion/arthrodesis along these segments

13. After appropriate hemostasis is obtained, muscle and skin incisions can then be closed in appropriate fashion, often with placement of postoperative drains that can be removed after 2 to 3 days

## Surgical Procedure for Anterior Cervical Spine

1. Informed consent signed, preoperative labs normal, no Aspirin/Plavix/Coumadin/NSAIDs/Celebrex/Naprosyn/other anticoagulants and anti-inflammatory drugs for at least 2 weeks

2. Appropriate intubation and sedation and lines (if necessary) as per the anesthetist

3. Patient placed in supine position, breathing through endotracheal tube with ventilator

4. Neuromonitoring may be required to monitor nerves

5. Time out is performed with agreement from everyone in the room for correct patient and correct surgery with consent signed

6. Make a 2 to 4 cm (about 1 inch) transverse neck crease incision at the appropriate level off of the midline

7. Incise fascia over the platysma muscle and split it into a superficial plane in line with the neck incision

8. Identify anterior border of sternocleidomastoid muscle and incise fascia to retract it laterally

9. Identify and retract strap muscles medially (sternohyoid and sternothyroid), forming another middle plane
   a. The plane between the sternocleidomastoid muscle and the strap muscles can now be entered
   b. A plane between the esophagus and the carotid sheath will be created next for entry

10. Identify the carotid pulse and retract carotid sheath laterally

11. Cut through the pretracheal fascia

12. Localize superior and inferior thyroid arteries, tying them off if necessary
13. Split longus colli muscles and anterior longitudinal ligament
14. Subperiosteally dissect to identify anterior vertebral body, utilizing retractors and an operating microscope
15. Retract longus colli muscles laterally, forming a deep plane
16. Dissect thin layer of fibrous tissue covering vertebra away from disk space
17. Once the bone is exposed, it is best to localize and verify the correct vertebra via X-ray or fluoroscopic imaging and confirming with at least two people in the room
18. Perform the diskectomy over segments needed based on preoperative imaging of levels that are compressed due to tumor:
    a. Using Leksell rongeurs and hand-held high-speed drill, remove the appropriate disk(s) or perform a complete corpectomy for added exposure
    b. Identify location of tumor and resect tumor as needed if epidural or within the spinal canal/cord (with care not to injure the vertebral artery)
        i. Use operative microscope and open the spinal cord dura midline with 11 blade and tack up the dural leaflets with suture (see ▶ Fig. 1.24)
        ii. If tumor is intradural and extramedullary, the tumor can then be resected carefully with microdissection technique without cord injury (neuromonitoring needed in these cases)
        iii. If tumor is intradural and intramedullary, with microdissection technique the cord must be entered midline and the tumor must be identified and resected starting centrally first, then around the edges (neuromonitoring needed in these cases)
19. After appropriate tumor resection, there may be need for additional stabilization to prevent kyphosis if the resection caused multiple segment decompression. Therefore, instrumentation with anterior cage and plate can be performed.
20. After appropriate hemostasis is obtained, muscle and skin incisions can then be closed in appropriate fashion, often with placement of postoperative drains that can be removed after 2 to 3 days

## Pitfalls

- Loss of neck mobility (minimal, unless fusion extended to occiput and C1)
- Intraoperative CSF leak
- Blood clot (deep vein thrombosis, or more severe pulmonary embolism)
- Damage to spinal nerves and/or cord

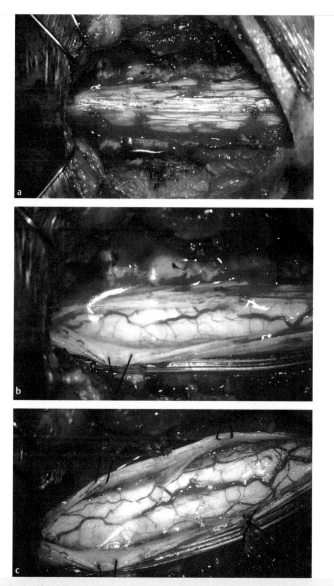

**Fig. 1.24 (a–c)** Intraoperative image of surgical exposure for cervical midline intra-medullary tumor resection. A laminoplasty was performed beforehand to visualize the dura. (Source: Operative considerations and surgical pearls. In: Baaj A, Kakaria U, Kim H, eds. Surgery of the Thoracic Spine: Principles and Techniques. 1st ed. Thieme; 2019).

- Postoperative weakness or numbness or continued pain
- Postoperative wound infection
- Continued symptoms postsurgically/unresolved symptoms with no improvement to quality of life
- Prolonged hospitalization due to invasiveness of surgery and other comorbidities/iatrogenic infection
- Injury to trachea or esophagus (from anterior approach)
- Injury to vertebral or carotid arteries

## Prognosis

- Hospitalization rates depend on the type of procedure performed, preoperative examination status, and patient's age/comorbidities
- PT and OT will be needed postoperatively, immediately and as outpatient to regain strength
- Brace/Collar is used for 8 weeks after discharge to immobilize to increase rate of healing

# Bibliography

Rangel-Castilla L, Russin JJ, Zaidi HA, et al. Contemporary management of spinal AVFs and AVMs: lessons learned from 110 cases. Neurosurg Focus 2014;37(3):E14

# 2 Thoracic

*Christ Ordookhanian and Paul E. Kaloostian*

## 2.1 Trauma

### 2.1.1 Thoracic Decompression/Thoracic Fusion

#### Symptoms and Signs

- Chest tenderness and ecchymoses
- Paraplegia
- Diminished control of bowel/bladder function
- Moderate/severe back pain
- Respiratory distress
- Difficulty maintaining balance and walking
- Loss of sensation in hands
- Inability to conduct fine motor skills with hands

#### Surgical Pathology

- Thoracic spine benign/malignant trauma

#### Diagnostic Modalities:

- CT thoracic spine
- MRI thoracic spine
- CT or X-ray chest
- Ultrasonography

#### Differential Diagnosis

- Blunt trauma (complete and incomplete Spinal cord injury [SCI])
  - Pneumohemothorax, pulmonary contusion, cardiac contusion
- Penetrating trauma (complete and incomplete SCI)
- Wedge/compression fracture
- Burst fracture
- Chance fracture
- Fracture-dislocation

## Treatment Options

- Acute pain control with medications and pain management
- Physical therapy and rehabilitation
- If symptomatic with cord compression:
  - Urgent surgical decompression and fusion over implicated segments if deemed suitable candidate for surgery
  - If poor surgical candidate with poor life expectancy, medical management recommended
  - Surgery may be done anteriorly, posteriorly, or combined two-stage approach for added stabilization
  - May include a combination of the following techniques: Laminectomy (entire lamina, thickened ligaments, and part of enlarged facet joints removed to relieve pressure), Laminotomy (section of lamina and ligament removed), Foraminotomy (expanding space of neural foramen by removing soft tissues, small disk fragments, and bony spurs in the locus), Laminoplasty (expanding space within spinal canal by repositioning lamina), Diskectomy (removal of section of herniated disk), Corpectomy (removal of vertebral body and disks), Bony Spur Removal

## Indications for Surgical Intervention

- Spinal stenosis
- No improvement after nonoperative therapy (physical therapy, pain management)
- Partial paraplegia
- Residual spinal compression (see ▶ Fig. 2.1)
- Existence of blunt chest trauma or potential hemorrhagic lesions
- Unstable patterns of fracture
- Sufficient disruption of supporting ligaments

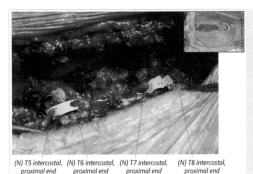

(N) T5 intercostal, proximal end   (N) T6 intercostal, proximal end   (N) T7 intercostal, proximal end   (N) T8 intercostal, proximal end

**Fig. 2.1** A patient with thoracic trauma and cord compression received decompression of the intercostal nerves (T5–T8). After decompression was achieved, the nerves were transected in preparation for nerve looping. (Source: Patient 12. In: Mackinnon S, ed. Nerve Surgery. 1st ed. Thieme; 2015).

# Surgical Procedure for Posterior Thoracic Spine

1. Informed consent signed, preoperative labs normal, no Aspirin/Plavix/Coumadin/NSAIDs/Advil/Celebrex/Ibuprofen/Motrin/Naprosyn/Aleve/other anticoagulants and anti-inflammatory drugs for at least 2 weeks
2. Appropriate intubation and sedation and lines (if necessary) as per the anesthetist
3. Patient placed prone on Jackson Table with all pressure points padded
4. Neuromonitoring may be required to monitor nerves (if necessary and indicated)
5. Time out is performed with agreement from everyone in the room for correct patient and correct surgery with consent signed
6. Make an incision down the midline of back
7. Subperiosteal dissection of muscles bilaterally exposing the spinous process and paraspinal muscles
8. Dissect tissue planes along spinous process and laminae using rongeurs
9. Move paraspinal muscles laterally to expose the laminae
10. Once the locus of interest is exposed, it is best to localize and verify the correct vertebra via X-ray or fluoroscopic imaging and confirming with at least two people in the room
11. Perform the decompression procedure over segments needed based on preoperative imaging of levels that are compressed due to trauma:
    a. Using Leksell rongeurs and hand-held high-speed drill, remove the bony spinous process and bilateral lamina as indicated for specific procedure (laminectomy)
    b. Or, remove bone of lamina above and below spinal nerves to create a small opening of lamina, relieving compression (laminotomy)
    c. If compression is diagnosed to be from spondylolisthesis, a diskectomy is performed (remove portion of slipped disk)
    d. Remove the thick ligamentum flavum and any bone spurs with Kerrison rongeurs with careful dissection beneath the ligament to ensure no adhesions exist to dura mater below and thus avoiding cerebrospinal fluid (CSF) leak
    e. Perform appropriate foraminotomy with Kerrison rongeurs as needed for appropriate decompression of nerve roots
12. Perform spinal fusion with instrumentation (often needed in trauma cases):
    a. Place pedicle screws over segments involved with connecting rods bilaterally, in addition to bone grafting, to fuse these segments (see ▶ Fig. 2.2 and Fig. 2.3)
13. After appropriate hemostasis is obtained, muscle and skin incisions can then be closed in appropriate fashion, often with placement of postoperative drains that can be removed after 2 to 3 days

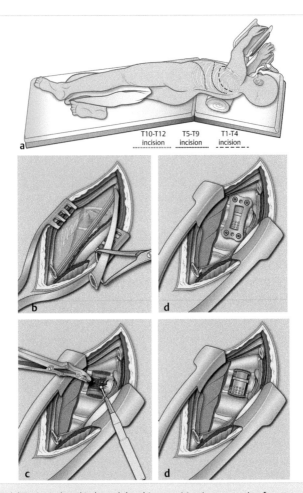

Fig. 2.2 (a) Patient placed in lateral decubitus position in preparation for a transthoracic vertebrectomy approach for decompression and fusion in response to thoracic trauma. Dashed lines represent levels of incision for the following thoracic segments: T10–T12, T5–T9, and T1–T4. (b) For dissection, electrocautery is employed to transect muscle. The rib is visualized and resected. After visualizing the neurovascular bundle, ligate and cut it. (c) The vertebrectomy is performed by removing the vertebral body and the surrounding disks with a drill and Kerrison rongeurs. Avoid damage to the thecal sac for decompression. (d) Following vertebrectomy, fusion is performed with instrumentation for stabilization. An autograft, allograft, or cage may be used. Place a plate and screws for proper fixation. (Source: Operative procedure. In: Ullman J, Raksin P, eds. Atlas of Emergency Neurosurgery. 1st ed. Thieme; 2015).

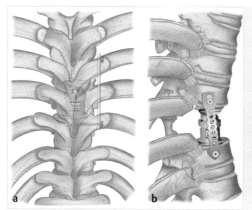

**Fig. 2.3 (a, b)** Illustration of thoracic fusion and instrumentation with an expandable cage in a thoracic trauma patient. Fusion was preceded by a thoracic corpectomy. (Source: Anterior thoracic arthrodesis after corpectomy (expandable cages, metallic mesh cages). In: Vaccaro A, Albert T, eds. Spine Surgery: Tricks of the Trade. 3rd eds. Thieme; 2016).

## Pitfalls

- Reduction in range of motion and mobility of fused spinal segments
- Intraoperative CSF leak
- Blood clot (deep vein thrombosis, or more severe pulmonary embolism)
- Damage to spinal nerves and/or cord
- Postoperative weakness or numbness or continued pain
- Postoperative wound infection
- Continued symptoms postsurgically/unresolved symptoms with no improvement to quality of life
- Prolonged hospitalization due to invasiveness of surgery and other comorbidities/iatrogenic infection
- Loss of sensation
- Progressive kyphosis
- Residual spinal compression
- Problems with bowel/bladder control

## Prognosis

- Hospitalization rates depend on the type of procedure performed, preoperative examination status, and patient's age/comorbidities
- Pain medications for postsurgical pain
- Catheter placed in bladder and removed 1 to 2 days postsurgery
- Physical therapy and occupational therapy will be needed postoperatively, immediately and as outpatient to regain strength
- Brace placed after discharge to immobilize to increase the rate of healing

## 2.1.2 Thoracic Corpectomy and Fusion

### Symptoms and Signs

- Chest tenderness and ecchymoses
- Paraplegia
- Diminished control of bowel/bladder function
- Moderate/severe back pain
- Respiratory distress
- Difficulty maintaining balance and walking
- Loss of sensation in hands
- Inability to conduct fine motor skills with hands
- Pain, weakness, numbness on either side of back, chest, or from bicep to wrist of one arm

### Surgical Pathology

- Thoracic spine benign/malignant trauma

### Diagnostic Modalities

- CT thoracic spine
- MRI thoracic spine
- CT or X-ray chest
- Ultrasonography

### Differential Diagnosis

- Blunt trauma (complete and incomplete SCI)
    - Pneumohemothorax, pulmonary contusion, cardiac contusion
- Penetrating trauma (complete and incomplete SCI)
- Wedge/Compression fracture
- Burst fracture
- Chance fracture
- Fracture-dislocation

### Treatment Options

- Acute pain control with medications and pain management
- Physical therapy and rehabilitation
- If symptomatic with cord compression:
    - Urgent surgical decompression and fusion over implicated segments if deemed suitable candidate for surgery

- If poor surgical candidate with poor life expectancy, medical management recommended
  - Surgery may be done anteriorly, posteriorly, or combined two-stage approach for added stabilization
  - May include a combination of the following techniques: Laminectomy (entire lamina, thickened ligaments, and part of enlarged facet joints removed to relieve pressure), Laminotomy (section of lamina and ligament removed), Foraminotomy (expanding space of neural foramen by removing soft tissues, small disk fragments, and bony spurs in the locus), Laminoplasty (expanding space within spinal canal by repositioning lamina), Diskectomy (removal of section of herniated disk), Corpectomy (removal of vertebral body and disks), Bony Spur Removal
- Corpectomy approaches:
  - Anterior (Thoracoscopic): Pleural entry to access anterior thoracic; broadest canal decompression, satisfactory visualization of thecal sac; easy graft insertion; anterolateral screw-plate fixation (see ▶ Fig. 2.4 and ▶ Fig. 2.5)
  - Anterolateral (Retropleural): Most direct anterior approach requiring retropleural dissection; canal decompression; anterolateral screw-plate fixation
  - Posterolateral (Lateral Extracavitary): Satisfactory visualization of thecal sac; anterior stabilization; posterior tension band preservation; unilateral decompression (see ▶ Fig. 2.6)
  - Posterior (Transpedicular): Circumferential decompression; difficult graft insertion; unideal thecal sac positioning (see ▶ Fig. 2.7)

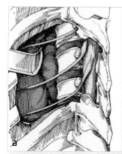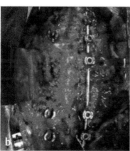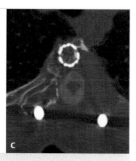

**Fig. 2.4 (a–c)** Posterolateral approach to performing a cervicothoracic corpectomy. Illustration demonstrates operative view. Intraoperative image demonstrates exposure for multilevel thoracic corpectomy, and postoperative CT scan demonstrates successful corpectomy from a unilateral approach. (Source: Cervicothoracic corpectomy. In: Fessler R, Sekhar L, eds. Atlas of Neurosurgical Techniques: Spine and Peripheral Nerves. 2nd ed. Thieme; 2016).

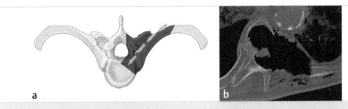

**Fig. 2.5 (a, b)** Illustration demonstrates trajectory of thoracic corpectomy, from a posterior approach, as well as the area of bone removal (colored). Postoperative CT scan demonstrates successful thoracic corpectomy. (Source: Procedure. In: Kim D, Choi G, Lee S, et al, eds. Endoscopic Spine Surgery. 2nd ed. Thieme; 2018).

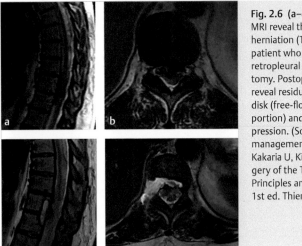

**Fig. 2.6 (a–d)** Preoperative MRI reveal thoracic disk herniation (T7–T8) in a patient who received lateral, retropleural partial corpectomy. Postoperative MRI reveal residual intradural disk (free-floating calcified portion) and cord decompression. (Source: Surgical management. In: Baaj A, Kakaria U, Kim H, eds. Surgery of the Thoracic Spine: Principles and Techniques. 1st ed. Thieme; 2019).

## Indications for Surgical Intervention

- Spinal stenosis
- No improvement after nonoperative therapy (physical therapy, pain management)
- Partial paraplegia
- Progressive cord compression
- Progressive kyphosis/deformity
- Existence of blunt chest trauma or potential hemorrhagic lesions
- Unstable patterns of fracture
- Sufficient disruption of supporting ligaments
- Compression places thoracic spine at risk of permanent damage

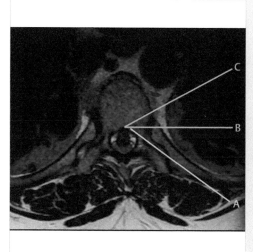

**Fig. 2.7** Surgical trajectories to addressing a thoracic disk herniation (image demonstrates giant calcified herniation in central canal). Line A is a costotransversectomy approach, Line B is a lateral transthoracic/retropleural approach, and Line C is an anterior transthoracic approach. Both transthoracic approaches do not require cord retraction. (Source: Surgical management. In: Baaj A, Kakaria U, Kim H, eds. Surgery of the Thoracic Spine: Principles and Techniques. 1st ed. Thieme; 2019).

## Surgical Procedure for Retropleural Thoracic Corpectomy

1. Informed consent signed, preoperative labs normal, no Aspirin/Plavix/Coumadin/NSAIDs/Advil/Celebrex/Ibuprofen/Motrin/Naprosyn/Aleve/other anticoagulants and anti-inflammatory drugs for at least 2 weeks
2. Appropriate intubation and sedation and lines (if necessary) as per the anesthetist
3. Patient placed in left/right lateral decubitus position with padding of upper and lower extremities, held in place with tape over upper and lower extremities
4. Fluoroscopy is used to confirm that no vertebral movement has occurred
5. Neuromonitoring may be required to monitor nerves (if necessary and indicated)
6. Time out is performed with agreement from everyone in the room for correct patient and correct surgery with consent signed
7. Make 6 cm incision from posterior axillary line to 4 cm lateral of midline
8. Dissect toward the rib head:
   a. Perform rib resection
   b. Incise endothoracic fascia, dissecting off the parietal pleura
   c. Dissect areolar tissue until endothoracic fascia is opened over rib head
9. Take down costovertebral ligaments and proximal rib head, exposing vertebral body

10. Perform corpectomy in a pedicle-to-pedicle fashion, preserving anterior shell of bone and anterior longitudinal ligament:
    a. Using hand-held curved high-speed drill, remove the posterior wall of vertebral bodies
    b. Remove the vertebral bodies and disks associated with the trauma
    c. Introduce hemostatic agents, if necessary, to control bleeding
    d. Achieve hemostasis
11. Perform spinal fusion
    a. Perform reconstruction with expandable cage and autograft
    b. Perform ventrolateral screw-plate fixation
    c. Perform midline posterior incision and place posterior percutaneous screws
12. Place chest tube if significant pleural tear occurs (can be removed in 2–3 days)
13. Remove retractor and inspect wound for further bleeding and pleural violations
14. Place red rubber catheter between endothoracic fascia and parietal pleura
15. Close fascia with suture
16. Catheter under water seal; the patient is made to valsalva with help of anesthesia
17. Remove catheter and tighten last facial suture
18. Close the muscle, subcutaneous layers, and skin

## Surgical Procedure for Lateral Extracavitary Thoracic Corpectomy

1. Informed consent signed, preoperative labs normal, no Aspirin/Plavix/Coumadin/NSAIDs/Advil/Celebrex/Ibuprofen/Motrin/Naprosyn/Aleve/other anticoagulants and anti-inflammatory drugs for at least 2 weeks
2. Appropriate intubation and sedation and lines (if necessary) as per the anesthetist
3. Patient placed prone on Jackson Table with all pressure points padded
4. Neuromonitoring may be required to monitor nerves (if necessary and indicated)
5. Time out is performed with agreement from everyone in the room for correct patient and correct surgery with consent signed
6. Make 4 cm incision, 4 cm laterally from midline
7. Remove proximal rib, costovertebral ligaments, rib head, intercostal vessels, and ipsilateral pedicle
8. Perform corpectomy, preserving ventral body, anterior longitudinal ligament, and contralateral vertebral margins:
    a. Using hand-held curved high-speed drill, remove the posterior wall of vertebral bodies

b. Remove the vertebral bodies and disks associated with the trauma
c. Introduce hemostatic agents, if necessary, to control bleeding
d. Achieve hemostasis

9. Perform spinal fusion:
   a. Perform reconstruction using titanium mesh, autograft, and/or expandable cages
      i. Supplement with vertebral body screws and rods if deemed necessary
   b. Place posterior percutaneous screws and rods above and below the level of corpectomy
10. Place chest tube if significant pleural tear occurs (can be removed in 2–3 days)
11. Remove retractor and inspect wound for further bleeding
12. After appropriate hemostasis is obtained, muscle and skin incisions can then be closed in appropriate fashion

## Surgical Procedure for Transpedicular Thoracic Corpectomy

1. Informed consent signed, preoperative labs normal, no Aspirin/Plavix/Coumadin/NSAIDs/Advil/Celebrex/Ibuprofen/Motrin/Naprosyn/Aleve/other anticoagulants and anti-inflammatory drugs for at least 2 weeks
2. Appropriate intubation and sedation and lines (if necessary) as per the anesthetist
3. Patient placed prone on Jackson Table with all pressure points padded
4. Neuromonitoring may be required to monitor nerves (if necessary and indicated)
5. Time out is performed with agreement from everyone in the room for correct patient and correct surgery with consent signed
6. C-arm fluoroscopy equipment set up in operation zone
7. Make midline incision two levels above and below the level of trauma, preserving the fascia
8. Perform dissection to lateral edge of transverse processes
9. Remove posterior elements and bilateral facets, exposing thecal sac and pedicles
10. Remove pedicles with drill, exposing vertebral body bilaterally
11. Perform corpectomy:
    a. Using Pituitary rongeurs and hand-held curved high-speed drill, remove the posterior wall of vertebral bodies
    b. Remove the vertebral bodies and disks associated with the trauma
    c. Introduce hemostatic agents, if necessary, to control bleeding
    d. Achieve hemostasis
12. Place posterior pedicle screws and rods two levels above and below the level of corpectomy

13. After appropriate hemostasis is obtained, muscle and skin incisions can then be closed in appropriate fashion

## Pitfalls

- Reduction in range of motion and mobility of fused spinal segments
- Intraoperative CSF leak
- Blood clot (deep vein thrombosis, or more severe pulmonary embolism)
- Damage to spinal nerves and/or cord
- Postoperative weakness or numbness or continued pain
- Postoperative wound infection
- Continued symptoms postsurgically/unresolved symptoms with no improvement to quality of life
- Prolonged hospitalization due to invasiveness of surgery and other comorbidities/iatrogenic infection
- Loss of sensation
- Progressive kyphosis
- Residual spinal compression
- Problems with bowel/bladder control
- Pulmonary contusion, atelectasis, pleural effusion, chylothorax, hemothorax
- Lumbar plexus damage, segmental artery damage
- Muscle dissection-related morbidity
- Pleural damage

## Prognosis

- Hospitalization rates depend on the type of procedure performed, preoperative examination status, and patient's age/comorbidities
- Pain medications for postsurgical pain
- Catheter placed in bladder and removed 1 to 2 days after surgery
- Physical therapy and occupational therapy will be needed postoperatively as outpatient to regain strength
- External back brace placed after discharge

## 2.1.3 Transthoracic Approaches for Decompression and Fusion/Transsternal Approaches for Decompression and Fusion

### Symptoms and Signs

- Chest tenderness and ecchymoses
- Paraplegia

- Diminished control of bowel/bladder function
- Moderate/severe back pain
- Respiratory distress
- Difficulty maintaining balance and walking
- Loss of sensation in hands
- Inability to conduct fine motor skills with hands
- Trachea deviates away from side of tension pneumothorax

## Surgical Pathology

- Thoracic spine benign/malignant trauma

## Diagnostic Modalities

- CT thoracic spine
- MRI thoracic spine
- CT or X-ray chest
- Ultrasonography

## Differential Diagnosis

- Blunt trauma (complete and incomplete SCI)
  - Pneumohemothorax, pulmonary contusion, cardiac contusion
- Penetrating trauma (complete and incomplete SCI)
- Wedge/Compression fracture
- Burst fracture
- Chance fracture
- Fracture-dislocation

## Treatment Options

- Acute pain control with medications and pain management
- Physical therapy and rehabilitation
- If symptomatic with cord compression:
  - Urgent surgical decompression and fusion over implicated segments if deemed suitable candidate for surgery
  - If poor surgical candidate with poor life expectancy, medical management recommended
  - Surgery may be done anteriorly, posteriorly, or combined two-stage approach for added stabilization
  - May include a combination of the following techniques: Laminectomy (entire lamina, thickened ligaments, and part of enlarged facet joints removed to relieve pressure), Laminotomy (section of lamina and

ligament removed), Foraminotomy (expanding space of neural foramen by removing soft tissues, small disk fragments, and bony spurs in the locus), Laminoplasty (expanding space within spinal canal by repositioning lamina), Diskectomy (removal of section of herniated disk), Corpectomy (removal of vertebral body and disks), Bony Spur Removal
  – Thoracic Decompression/Fusion Approaches:
- Anterior transthoracic (see ▶ Fig. 2.8):
  – Excellent exposure to anterior thoracic spine, vertebral bodies, intervertebral disks, spinal canal, and nerve roots
  – Posterior elements and contralateral pedicle inaccessible
  – No extensive bone resection or corpectomy
  – Can freely use hemostatic agents in locus of bone removal since lateral fusion is performed
  – Do not perform if there is displacement of posterior bone elements into spinal canal or when posterior penetrating injury exists (unless as part of a combined procedure)
  – T2–T9 is preferentially approached from the right side to avoid injury to heart, aortic arch, and great vessels

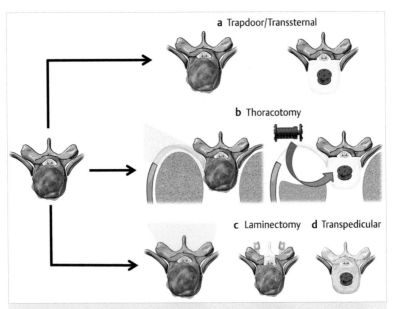

**Fig. 2.8** Illustration of different approaches to the thoracic spine. The transsternal approach allows anterior access to the upper thoracic. (Source: Thoracic spine. In: Vialle L, ed. AOSpine Masters Series, Volume 1: Metastatic Spinal Tumors. 1st ed. Thieme; 2014).

- T10–L2 is preferentially approached from the left side to avoid injury to liver
- Anterior transsternal (see ▶ Fig. 2.9):
  - Direct anterior exposure of thoracic spine
  - Excellent for upper thoracic access and cervicothoracic exposure

## Indications for Surgical Intervention

- Spinal stenosis
- No improvement after nonoperative therapy (physical therapy, pain management)
- Partial paraplegia
- Residual spinal compression
- Existence of blunt chest trauma or potential hemorrhagic lesions
- Unstable patterns of fracture
- Sufficient disruption of supporting ligaments
- Transthoracic/Transsternal approaches:
  - Partial injury of thoracic cord
  - Anterior compression
  - No intraspinal displacement of posterior bone elements
  - Anterior spinal cord syndrome with partial or complete myelographic spinal block
  - Thoracic disk disease
  - Vertebral osteomyelitis of diskitis

## Surgical Procedure for Anterior Transthoracic Decompression/Fusion

1. Informed consent signed, preoperative labs normal, no Aspirin/Plavix/Coumadin/NSAIDs/Advil/Celebrex/Ibuprofen/Motrin/Naprosyn/Aleve/other anticoagulants and anti-inflammatory drugs for at least 2 weeks
2. Appropriate intubation and sedation and lines (if necessary) as per the anesthetist
3. Large bore (16–14 gauge) intravenous (IV) access for blood loss during operation
4. Patient placed in left/right lateral decubitus position with all pressure points padded (depending on whether left or right lateral thoracotomy will be performed)
5. Neuromonitoring may be required to monitor nerves (if necessary and indicated)
6. Intraoperative fluoroscopy used as deemed appropriate

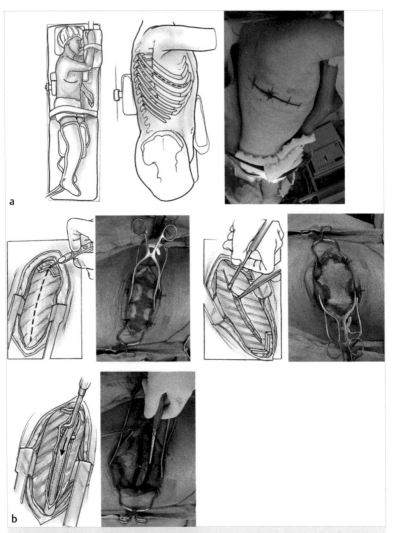

**Fig. 2.9** **(a)** Patient orientation for the anterolateral transthoracic approach to thoracic decompression and fusion. **(b)** Surgical steps for anterolateral transthoracic approach, from incision and retractor placement to muscular dissection, rib visualization, electrocautery, and rib resection.

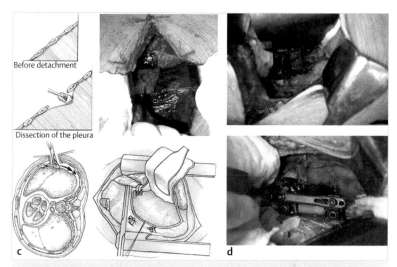

**Fig. 2.9** (*Continued*) (**c**) Following initial thoracotomy, either retropleural or transpleural approaches are viable. This image demonstrates the next steps in a retropleural approach. (**d**) Intraoperative image of a lateral transthoracic approach to a thoracic vertebrectomy and fusion with instrumentation. (Source: Open lateral transthoracic approach. In: Fessler R, Sekhar L, eds. Atlas of Neurosurgical Techniques: Spine and Peripheral Nerves. 2nd ed. Thieme; 2016).

7. Time out is performed with agreement from everyone in the room for correct patient and correct surgery with consent signed
8. Make posterior incision starting from appropriate level of spine, curving down the line of the rib
9. Divide the latissimus and trapezius muscles:
    a. Divide the rhomboids and both teres as well for T1–T4 exposure
10. Mobilize scapula from chest wall and elevate using scapula retractor
11. Enter chest through intercostal space or the bed of the rib at the level of vertebrae of interest:
    a. Make incision in intercostal space to enter thoracic cavity
    b. Resect proximal rib as bone graft will be used
    c. Mobilize erector spinae superiorly and inferiorly, or divide it transversely at the level of intercostal incision
    d. Retract ribs and scapula using Finochietto or Burford retractor
    e. Retract the intercostal space

12. Expose the vertebrae of interest:
    a. Mobilize superior and posterior hilum (T1–T4)
    b. Mobilize the pulmonary ligament and hilar pleura
    c. Divide the mediastinal pleura posterior to the hilum from the inferior pulmonary vein to just above the mainstem bronchus (T5–T8)
    d. Displace the lung anteriorly and move it out of the way using wet lap pads
    e. Open the mediastinal pleura anterior to the vertebral bodies vertically from the thoracic inlet to the level of the carina. Dissect and mobilize the mediastinal structures. Mobilize the azygos vein with tributaries and the esophagus using blunt and sharp dissection (right thoracotomy), or mobilize the descending thoracic aorta (left thoracotomy) (T1–T8)
    f. Mobilize the thoracic duct anteriorly (T5–T8)
    g. Retract diaphragm using sponge stick. Mobilize posterior attachments of diaphragm. Mobilize posterior mediastinal structures for anterior retraction (T9–T12)
13. Perform the decompression procedure over the desired segments based on preoperative imaging of levels that are compressed due to trauma:
    a. Using Leksell rongeurs and hand-held high-speed air drill, resect the adjacent disk material immediately ventral to the posterior cortical bone of the vertebral bodies
    b. Leave a thin shelf of bone immediately adjacent to posterior longitudinal ligament and dura intact:
        i. This step avoids the cord falling ventrally, which can result in cord injury during the resection process
    c. Remove adequate portion of subcortical bone, using high-speed air drill, across midline for decompression of ventral cord surface
    d. Remove thin shelf of bone adjacent to posterior longitudinal ligament with rongeur
    e. Control bone bleeding with bone wax
14. Perform posterior thoracic fusion with instrumentation (if necessary, as most often anterior approach is all that is needed):
    a. Place and secure bone graft with cancellous screws to bridge the vertebra above and below the midpoint of the fracture, avoiding injury to vital structures
15. Achieve hemostasis
16. Drain the chest and inspect posterior mediastinum for lymph leak
17. If previously mobilized, reattach the diaphragm to the fascia of the posterior chest wall with sutures
18. Close muscle and skin incisions in appropriate fashion, often with placement of postoperative chest tube that can be removed after 2 to 3 days

# Surgical Procedure Anterior Transsternal Decompression/Fusion

1. Informed consent signed, preoperative labs normal, no Aspirin/Plavix/Coumadin/NSAIDs/Advil/Celebrex/Ibuprofen/Motrin/Naprosyn/Aleve/other anticoagulants and anti-inflammatory drugs for at least 2 weeks
2. Appropriate intubation and sedation and lines (if necessary) as per the anesthetist
3. Patient placed in supine position with all pressure points padded
4. Neuromonitoring may be required to monitor nerves (if necessary and indicated)
5. Time out is performed with agreement from everyone in the room for correct patient and correct surgery with consent signed
6. Make an incision on medial border of right sternocleidomastoid, extending down over manubrium
7. Perform median sternotomy with sternal saw (see ▶ Fig. 2.10)
8. Mobilize sternocleidomastoid laterally and trachea/esophagus medially, exposing anterior cervicothoracic spine
9. Perform the decompression procedure over the desired segments based on preoperative imaging of levels that are compressed due to trauma:
   a. Using Leksell rongeurs and hand-held high-speed drill, remove disk material at the affected level
   b. Remove the thick ligamentum and any bone spurs with Kerrison rongeurs with careful dissection beneath the ligament to ensure no adhesions exist to dura mater below and thus avoiding CSF leak

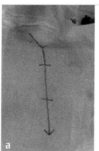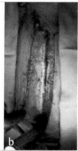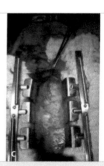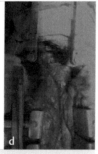

**Fig. 2.10** Intraoperative images demonstrating anterior cervicothoracic view. (**a, b**) Represent the incision position for a transsternal approach to a T1 corpectomy. (**c, d**) The exposure of the ventral cervicothoracic junction using retractors, following a sternotomy. (Source: Cervicothoracic corpectomy. In: Fessler R, Sekhar L, eds. Atlas of Neurosurgical Techniques: Spine and Peripheral Nerves. 2nd ed. Thieme; 2016).

    c. Perform complete decompression of anterior cord with Kerrison rongeurs as needed for appropriate decompression of nerve roots

    d. Irrigate surgical site

10. Perform spinal fusion with instrumentation (if necessary, most often not needed):

    a. Perform reconstruction with expandable cage and autograft

    b. Perform screw-plate fixation

11. After appropriate hemostasis is obtained, muscle and skin incisions can then be closed in appropriate fashion, often with placement of postoperative Jackson-Pratt drains:

    a. Achieve closure of sternum with sternal wires

## Pitfalls

- Reduction in range of motion and mobility of fused spinal segments
- Intraoperative CSF leak
- Blood clot (deep vein thrombosis, or more severe pulmonary embolism)
- Damage to spinal nerves and/or cord
- Postoperative weakness or numbness or continued pain
- Postoperative wound infection
- Continued symptoms postsurgically/unresolved symptoms with no improvement to quality of life
- Prolonged hospitalization due to invasiveness of surgery and other comorbidities/iatrogenic infection
- Loss of sensation
- Progressive kyphosis
- Residual spinal compression
- Problems with bowel/bladder control
- Injury to artery of Adamkiewicz (generally originating from the left T8–L1) resulting in cord ischemia, radicular arteries (typically during dissection around intervertebral foramina), thoracic duct, chylothorax, and/or esophagus (from transthoracic approach)
- Vascular complications
- Atelectasis and pneumonia
- Hemothorax and empyema (managed with drainage and antibiotics)
- Injury to carotid sheath, trachea, esophagus, recurrent laryngeal nerves, great vessels, vertebral arteries, and/or sympathetic trunk (from transsternal approach)

## Prognosis

- Hospitalization rates depend on the type of procedure performed, preoperative examination status, and patient's age/comorbidities

- Pain medications for postsurgical pain
- Catheter placed in bladder and removed 1 to 2 days after surgery
- Physical therapy and occupational therapy will be needed postoperatively as outpatient to regain strength
- Brace (i.e., Jewett or Taylor type) placed after discharge (patient can be mobilized after 2 to 3 weeks of transthoracic decompression/fusion operation)

# 2.2 Elective

## 2.2.1 Thoracic Decompression/Thoracic Fusion

### Symptoms and Signs

- Moderate back pain
- Muscle weakness and reduction of mobility from pain (as opposed to from nerve impairment, which typically requires emergent treatment, particularly if it relates to bladder function)
- Pain and discomfort derived from consistent nerve irritation
- Difficulty maintaining balance and walking
- Tingling numbness in arms/legs/hands
- Abnormal spinal curvature
- Spinal instability

### Surgical Pathology

- Thoracic spine benign/malignant trauma
- Thoracic spine benign/malignant tumor
- Thoracic vascular benign/malignant lesion

### Diagnostic Modalities

- Clinical examination
- CT of thoracic spine with and without contrast
- MRI of thoracic spine with and without contrast
- CT or X-ray chest
- Ultrasonography
- Angiography
- PET scan (search for tumor foci)
- Biopsy (determine severity of tumor and possible type of cancer)

### Differential Diagnosis

- Thoracic disk herniation
- Spinal stenosis (narrowing of the spine)

- Scoliosis
- Bulging thoracic disk
- Presence of bony spurs
- Tumor:
  - Metastatic (malignant, requiring emergent treatment)
  - Primary (benign or malignant)
- Vascular lesion (typically requiring supplemental embolization):
  - Fibromuscular dysplasia (FMD)
  - Spinal arteriovenous malformation (AVM)
  - Spinal dural arteriovenous fistula (AVF)
  - Thoracic outlet syndrome (TOS)
- Vertebral fracture:
  - Blunt trauma (incomplete SCI)
  - Penetrating trauma (incomplete SCI)
  - Wedge/compression fracture
  - Burst fracture
  - Chance fracture
  - Fracture-dislocation

## Treatment Options

- Acute pain control with medications and pain management
- Physical therapy and rehabilitation
- If asymptomatic or mildly symptomatic with pain/radiculopathy with small focus of tumor:
  - Radiation treatment (radiation oncology consultation)
  - Some metastatic tumors are radioresistant
  - Chemotherapy (medical oncology consultation)
  - Some metastatic tumors are radioresistant
  - Kyphoplasty (to treat pain)
  - Surgical instrumentation and fusion (if there is concern for deformity, instability, or cord compression)
- If asymptomatic or mildly symptomatic with thoracic cord compression:
  - Surgical decompression and fusion over implicated segments if deemed suitable candidate for surgery:
  - If poor surgical candidate with poor life expectancy, medical management recommended
  - Surgery may be done anteriorly, posteriorly, or combined two-stage approach for added stabilization
  - May include a combination of the following techniques: Laminectomy (entire lamina, thickened ligaments, and part of enlarged facet joints removed to relieve pressure), Laminotomy (section of lamina and ligament removed), Foraminotomy (expanding space of neural foramen by

removing soft tissues, small disk fragments, and bony spurs in the locus), Laminoplasty (expanding space within spinal canal by repositioning lamina), Diskectomy (removal of section of herniated disk), Corpectomy (removal of vertebral body and disks), Bony Spur Removal
- Approaches: Posterior, anterior transthoracic, anterior transsternal

## Indications for Surgical Intervention

- Spinal stenosis
- No sufficient improvement of pain and other symptoms after nonoperative measures (physical therapy, medications/injections, pain management)
- Thoracic compression
- Spinal condition isolated to specific locus of the body
- Significant reduction in everyday activities due to symptoms
- Expected postsurgical favorable outcome

## Surgical Procedure for Posterior Thoracic Spine

1. Informed consent signed, preoperative labs normal, no Aspirin/Plavix/ Coumadin/NSAIDs/Celebrex/Naprosyn/other anticoagulants and anti-inflammatory drugs for at least 2 weeks
2. Appropriate intubation and sedation and lines (if necessary) as per the anesthetist
3. Patient placed prone on Jackson Table with all pressure points padded
4. Neuromonitoring may be required to monitor nerves
5. Time out is performed with agreement from everyone in the room for correct patient and correct surgery with consent signed
6. Make an incision down the midline of back
7. Perform subperiosteal dissection of muscles bilaterally exposing the spinous process and paraspinal muscles
8. Dissect tissue planes along spinous process and laminae using rongeurs
9. Move paraspinal muscles laterally to expose the laminae
10. Once the locus of interest is exposed, it is best to localize and verify the correct vertebra via X-ray or fluoroscopic imaging and confirming with at least two people in the room
11. Perform the decompression procedure over the desired segments based on preoperative imaging of levels that are compressed due to trauma (see ▶ Fig. 2.11 to Fig. 2.14):
    a. Using Leksell rongeurs and hand-held high-speed drill, remove the bony spinous process and bilateral lamina as indicated for specific procedure (laminectomy)
    b. Or, remove bone of lamina above and below spinal nerves to create a small opening of lamina, relieving compression (laminotomy)

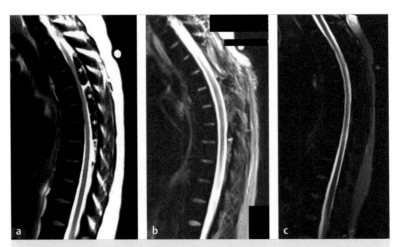

**Fig. 2.11** A middle-aged woman with a dorsal epidural lesion in T3–T8 and cord compression (**a**) received left T3–T5 hemilaminotomies and right T6–T8 hemilaminotomies, resecting the lesion (**b**). Follow-up MRI (1 year) demonstrates neither recurrence of lesion nor kyphosis (**c**). (Source: Minimally invasive thoracic decompression for multilevel thoracic pathology. In: Fessler R, Sekhar L, eds. Atlas of Neurosurgical Techniques: Spine and Peripheral Nerves. 2nd ed. Thieme; 2016).

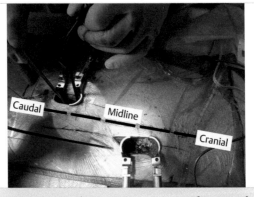

**Fig. 2.12** Intraoperative image demonstrating positioning of retractors for multilevel thoracic pathology. The retractors are expanded in the rostral–caudal direction. This is followed by electrocautery to visualize the lamina and achieve decompression. (Source: Minimally invasive thoracic decompression for multilevel thoracic pathology. In: Fessler R, Sekhar L, eds. Atlas of Neurosurgical Techniques: Spine and Peripheral Nerves. 2nd ed. Thieme; 2016).

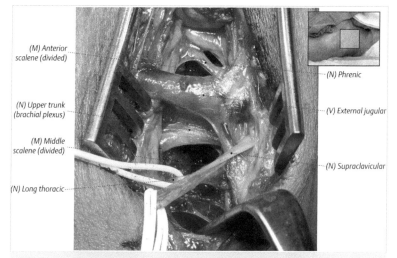

**Fig. 2.13** Image demonstrating relevant anatomy to thoracic outlet decompression. This anatomy is visualized after the anterior and middle scalene is divided, decompressing the brachial plexus. (Source: Authors' preferred technique. In: Mackinnon S, ed. Nerve Surgery. 1st ed. Thieme; 2015).

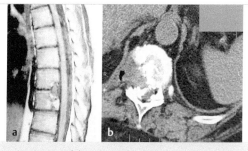

**Fig. 2.14** Postoperative MRI of thoracic reveals proper decompression of cord and spinal canal following a thoracoscopic diskectomy (**a**). Postoperative CT scan of thoracic reveals bony resection achieved during diskectomy (**b**). (Source: Technique for thoracoscopic diskectomy. In: Kim D, Choi G, Lee S, et al, eds. Endoscopic Spine Surgery. 2nd ed. Thieme; 2018).

    c. Remove the thick ligamentum flavum and any bone spurs with Kerrison rongeurs with careful dissection beneath the ligament to ensure no adhesions exist to dura mater below and thus avoiding CSF leak

    d. Perform appropriate foraminotomy with Kerrison rongeurs as needed for appropriate decompression of nerve roots

12. Perform spinal fusion with instrumentation:
    a. Place pedicle screws over two segments above and two segments below the problem level involved with connecting rods bilaterally, in addition to bone grafting, to fuse these segments
13. After appropriate hemostasis is obtained, muscle and skin incisions can then be closed in appropriate fashion, often with placement of postoperative drains that can be removed after 2 to 3 days

## Pitfalls

- Reduction in range of motion and mobility of fused spinal segments
- Intraoperative CSF leak
- Blood clot (deep vein thrombosis, or more severe pulmonary embolism)
- Damage to spinal nerves and/or cord
- Postoperative weakness or numbness or continued pain
- Postoperative wound infection
- Continued symptoms postsurgically/unresolved symptoms with no improvement to quality of life
- Prolonged hospitalization due to invasiveness of surgery and other comorbidities/iatrogenic infection
- Loss of sensation
- Progressive kyphosis
- Residual spinal compression
- Problems with bowel/bladder control

## Prognosis

- Hospitalization rates depend on the type of procedure performed, preoperative examination status, and patient's age/comorbidities.
- Pain medications for postsurgical pain.
- Catheter placed in bladder and removed 1 to 2 days after surgery
- Physical therapy and occupational therapy will be needed postoperatively, immediately and as outpatient to regain strength
- Brace placed after discharge to immobilize to increase rate of healing

# 2.2.2 Thoracic Corpectomy and Fusion

## Symptoms and Signs

- Moderate back pain
- Muscle weakness and reduction of mobility from pain (as opposed to from nerve impairment, which typically requires emergent treatment, particularly if it relates to bladder function)

- Pain and discomfort derived from consistent nerve irritation
- Difficulty maintaining balance and walking
- Tingling numbness in arms/legs/hands
- Abnormal spinal curvature
- Spinal instability

## Surgical Pathology

- Thoracic spine benign/malignant trauma
- Thoracic spine benign/malignant tumor
- Thoracic vascular benign/malignant lesion

## Diagnostic Modalities

- Clinical examination
- CT of thoracic spine with and without contrast
- MRI of thoracic spine with and without contrast
- CT or X-ray chest
- Ultrasonography
- Angiography
- PET scan (search for tumor foci)
- Biopsy (determine severity of tumor and possible type of cancer)

## Differential Diagnosis

- Thoracic disk herniation
- Spinal stenosis (narrowing of the spine)
- Scoliosis
- Bulging thoracic disk
- Presence of bony spurs
- Tumor:
  - Metastatic (malignant, requiring emergent treatment)
  - Primary (benign or malignant)
- Vascular lesion (typically requiring supplemental embolization): FMD
  - Spinal AVM
  - Spinal dural AVF TOS
- Vertebral fracture:
  - Blunt trauma (incomplete SCI)
  - Penetrating trauma (incomplete SCI)
  - Wedge/compression fracture
  - Burst fracture
  - Chance fracture
  - Fracture-dislocation

## Treatment Options

- Acute pain control with medications and pain management
- Physical therapy and rehabilitation
- If asymptomatic or mildly symptomatic with neck pain/radiculopathy with small focus of tumor:
  - Radiation treatment (radiation oncology consultation)
  - Some metastatic tumors are radioresistant
  - Chemotherapy (medical oncology consultation)
  - Some metastatic tumors are radioresistant
  - Kyphoplasty (to treat pain)
  - Surgical instrumentation and fusion (if there is concern for deformity, instability, or cord compression)
- If asymptomatic or mildly symptomatic with thoracic cord compression:
  - Surgical decompression and fusion over implicated segments if deemed suitable candidate for surgery
  - If poor surgical candidate with poor life expectancy, medical management recommended
  - Surgery may be done anteriorly, posteriorly, or combined two-stage approach for added stabilization
  - May include a combination of the following techniques: Laminectomy (entire lamina, thickened ligaments, and part of enlarged facet joints removed to relieve pressure), Laminotomy (section of lamina and ligament removed), Foraminotomy (expanding space of neural foramen by removing soft tissues, small disk fragments, and bony spurs in the locus), Laminoplasty (expanding space within spinal canal by repositioning lamina), Diskectomy (removal of section of herniated disk), Corpectomy (removal of vertebral body and disks), Bony Spur Removal
- Corpectomy Approaches:
  - Anterior (Thoracoscopic): Pleural entry to access anterior thoracic; broadest canal decompression, satisfactory visualization of thecal sac; easy graft insertion; anterolateral screw-plate fixation
  - Anterolateral (Retropleural): Most direct anterior approach requiring retropleural dissection; canal decompression; anterolateral screw-plate fixation
  - Posterolateral (Lateral Extracavitary): Satisfactory visualization of thecal sac; anterior stabilization; posterior tension band preservation; unilateral decompression
  - Posterior (Transpedicular): Circumferential decompression; difficult graft insertion; unideal thecal sac positioning

# Indications for Surgical Intervention

- Spinal stenosis
- No sufficient improvement of pain and other symptoms after nonoperative measures (physical therapy, medications/injections, pain management)
- Thoracic compression (see ▶ Fig. 2.15 and Fig. 2.16)
- Spinal condition isolated to specific locus of the body
- Significant reduction in everyday activities due to symptoms
- Expected postsurgical favorable outcome

# Surgical Procedure for Retropleural Thoracic Corpectomy

1. Informed consent signed, preoperative labs normal, no Aspirin/Plavix/Coumadin/NSAIDs/Celebrex/Naprosyn/other anticoagulants and anti-inflammatory drugs for at least 2 weeks
2. Appropriate intubation and sedation and lines (if necessary) as per the anesthetist
3. Patient placed in left/right lateral decubitus position with padding of upper and lower extremities, held in place with tape over upper and lower extremities
4. Fluoroscopy is used to confirm that no vertebral movement has occurred.
5. Neuromonitoring may be required to monitor nerves (if necessary and indicated)
6. Time out is performed with agreement from everyone in the room for correct patient and correct surgery with consent signed
7. Make 6 cm incision from posterior axillary line to 4 cm lateral of midline
8. Dissect toward the rib head:
   a. Perform rib resection
   b. Incise endothoracic fascia, dissecting off the parietal pleura
   c. Dissect areolar tissue until endothoracic fascia is opened over rib head
9. Take down costovertebral ligaments and proximal rib head, exposing vertebral body
10. Perform corpectomy in a pedicle-to-pedicle fashion at appropriate level, preserving anterior shell of bone and anterior longitudinal ligament:
    a. Using hand-held curved high-speed drill, remove the posterior wall of vertebral bodies
    b. Remove the vertebral bodies and disks associated with the trauma
    c. Introduce hemostatic agents, if necessary, to control bleeding
    d. Achieve hemostasis

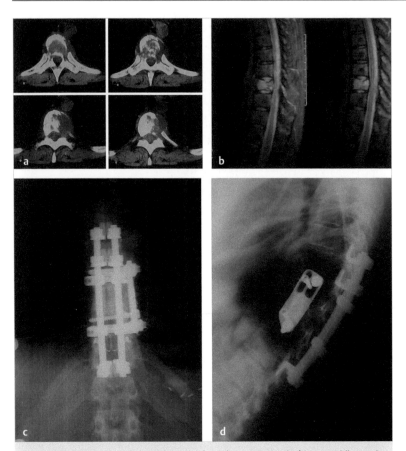

**Fig. 2.15** A CT scan revealed a T9 lesion with cord compression **(a, b)** in a middle-aged woman with a history of thoracic lymphomas. She received a left thoracotomy with anterior/posterior reconstruction and a T9 corpectomy and fusion with instrumentation **(c, d)**. (Source: Operative technique. In: Dickman C, Fehlings M, Gokaslan Z, eds. Spinal Cord and Spinal Column Tumors. 1st ed. Thieme; 2006).

11. Perform spinal fusion (see ▶ Fig. 2.17):
   a. Perform reconstruction with expandable cage and autograft
   b. Perform ventrolateral screw-plate fixation
   c. Perform midline posterior incision and place posterior percutaneous screws

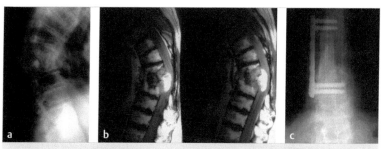

**Fig. 2.16** X-ray and MRI revealed thoracic kyphosis and compression (**a, b**) in an elderly man with a recurrent tumor and a history of thoracic chordomas. He received a left thoracotomy, a corpectomy (T6–T7), and an anterolateral fusion (T5–T8) with instrumentation (**c**). (Source: Operative technique. In: Dickman C, Fehlings M, Gokaslan Z, eds. Spinal Cord and Spinal Column Tumors. 1st ed. Thieme; 2006).

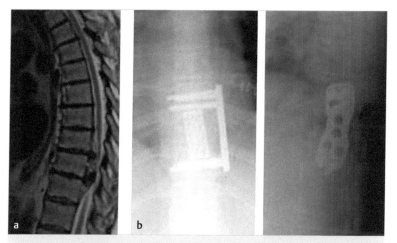

**Fig. 2.17** (**a, b**) A patient with thoracic myelopathy and a calcified disk received a thoracic corpectomy and fusion with instrumentation. (Source: Stabilization and reconstruction techniques for the thoracolumbar spine (fractures, tumors, degenerative). In: Aebi M, Arlet V, Webb J, eds. AOSPINE Manual: Principles and Techniques (Vol. 1). 1st ed. Thieme; 2007).

12. Place chest tube if significant pleural tear occurs (can be removed in 2–3 days)
13. Remove retractor and inspect wound for further bleeding and pleural violations

14. Place red rubber catheter between endothoracic fascia and parietal pleura
15. Close fascia with suture
16. Catheter under water seal; the patient is made to valsalva with help of anesthesia
17. Remove catheter and tighten last facial suture
18. Close the muscle, subcutaneous layers, and skin

## Surgical Procedure for Lateral Extracavitary Thoracic Corpectomy

1. Informed consent signed, preoperative labs normal, no Aspirin/Plavix/Coumadin/NSAIDs/Celebrex/Naprosyn/other anticoagulants and anti-inflammatory drugs for at least 2 weeks
2. Appropriate intubation and sedation and lines (if necessary) as per the anesthetist
3. Patient placed prone on Jackson Table with all pressure points padded
4. Neuromonitoring may be required to monitor nerves (if necessary and indicated)
5. Time out is performed with agreement from everyone in the room for correct patient and correct surgery with consent signed
6. Make 4 cm incision, 4 cm laterally from midline
7. Remove proximal rib, costovertebral ligaments, rib head, intercostal vessels, and ipsilateral pedicle
8. Perform corpectomy, preserving ventral body, anterior longitudinal ligament, and contralateral vertebral margins:
   a. Using hand-held curved high-speed drill, remove the posterior wall of vertebral bodies
   b. Remove the vertebral bodies and disks associated with the trauma
   c. Introduce hemostatic agents, if necessary, to control bleeding
   d. Achieve hemostasis
9. Perform spinal fusion:
   a. Perform reconstruction using titanium mesh, autograft, and/or expandable cages
      i. Supplement with vertebral body screws and rods if deemed necessary
   b. Place posterior percutaneous screws and rods above and below the level of corpectomy
10. Place chest tube if significant pleural tear occurs (can be removed in 2–3 days)
11. Remove retractor and inspect wound for further bleeding

12. After appropriate hemostasis is obtained, muscle and skin incisions can then be closed in appropriate fashion

## Surgical Procedure for Transpedicular Thoracic Corpectomy

1. Informed consent signed, preoperative labs normal, no Aspirin/Plavix/ Coumadin/NSAIDs/Celebrex/Naprosyn/other anticoagulants and anti-inflammatory drugs for at least 2 weeks
2. Appropriate intubation and sedation and lines (if necessary) as per the anesthetist
3. Patient placed prone on Jackson Table with all pressure points padded
4. Neuromonitoring may be required to monitor nerves (if necessary and indicated)
5. Time out is performed with agreement from everyone in the room for correct patient and correct surgery with consent signed
6. C-arm fluoroscopy equipment set up in operation zone
7. Make midline incision two levels above and below the level of trauma, preserving the fascia
8. Perform dissection to lateral edge of transverse processes
9. Remove posterior elements and bilateral facets, exposing thecal sac and pedicles
10. Remove pedicles with drill, thus exposing vertebral body bilaterally
11. Perform corpectomy:
    a. Using Pituitary rongeurs and hand-held curved high-speed drill, remove the posterior wall of vertebral bodies
    b. Remove the vertebral bodies and disks associated with the trauma
    c. Introduce hemostatic agents, if necessary, to control bleeding
    d. Achieve hemostasis
12. Place appropriate-sized cage and posterior screws and rods two levels above and below the level of corpectomy
13. After appropriate hemostasis is obtained, muscle and skin incisions can then be closed in appropriate fashion

## Pitfalls

- Reduction in range of motion and mobility of fused spinal segments
- Intraoperative CSF leak
- Blood clot (deep vein thrombosis, or more severe pulmonary embolism)
- Damage to spinal nerves and/or cord

- Postoperative weakness or numbness or continued pain
- Postoperative wound infection
- Continued symptoms postsurgically/unresolved symptoms with no improvement to quality of life
- Prolonged hospitalization due to invasiveness of surgery and other comorbidities/iatrogenic infection
- Loss of sensation
- Progressive kyphosis
- Residual spinal compression
- Problems with bowel/bladder control
- Pulmonary contusion, atelectasis, pleural effusion, chylothorax, hemothorax
- Lumbar plexus damage, segmental artery damage
- Muscle dissection-related morbidity
- Pleural damage

## Prognosis

- Hospitalization rates depend on the type of procedure performed, preoperative examination status, and patient's age/comorbidities
- After fusion, halt use of all NSAIDs for 6 months
- Can shower 1 to 4 days after surgery, based on surgeon's recommendation
- Pain medications for postsurgical pain
- Catheter placed in bladder and removed 1 to 2 days after surgery
- Physical therapy and occupational therapy will be needed postoperatively as outpatient to regain strength
- External back brace placed after discharge if necessary (up to 2 months, on a case-by-case basis)

## 2.2.3 Transthoracic Approaches for Decompression and Fusion/Transsternal Approaches for Decompression and Fusion

### Symptoms and Signs

- Moderate back pain
- Muscle weakness and reduction of mobility from pain (as opposed to from nerve impairment, which typically requires emergent treatment, particularly if it relates to bladder function)
- Pain and discomfort derived from consistent nerve irritation
- Difficulty maintaining balance and walking

- Tingling numbness in arms/legs/hands
- Abnormal spinal curvature
- Spinal instability

## Surgical Pathology

- Thoracic spine benign/malignant trauma
- Thoracic spine benign/malignant tumor
- Thoracic vascular benign/malignant lesion

## Diagnostic Modalities

- Clinical examination
- CT of thoracic spine with and without contrast
- MRI of thoracic spine with and without contrast
- CT or X-ray chest
- Ultrasonography
- Angiography
- PET scan (search for tumor foci)
- Biopsy (determine severity of tumor and possible type of cancer)

## Differential Diagnosis

- Thoracic disk herniation
- Spinal stenosis (narrowing of the spine)
- Scoliosis
- Bulging thoracic disk
- Presence of bony spurs
- Tumor:
  – Metastatic (malignant, requiring emergent treatment)
  – Primary (benign or malignant)
- Vascular lesion (typically requiring supplemental embolization): FMD
  – Spinal AVM
  – Spinal dural AVF TOS
- Vertebral fracture:
  – Blunt trauma (incomplete SCI)
  – Penetrating trauma (incomplete SCI)
  – Wedge/Compression fracture
  – Burst fracture
  – Chance fracture
  – Fracture-dislocation

## Treatment Options

- Acute pain control with medications and pain management
- Physical therapy and rehabilitation
- If asymptomatic or mildly symptomatic with neck pain/radiculopathy with small focus of tumor:
  - Radiation treatment (radiation oncology consultation)
  - Some metastatic tumors are radioresistant
  - Chemotherapy (medical oncology consultation)
  - Some metastatic tumors are radioresistant
  - Kyphoplasty (to treat pain)
  - Surgical instrumentation and fusion (if there is concern for deformity, instability, or cord compression)
- If asymptomatic or mildly symptomatic with thoracic cord compression:
  - Surgical decompression and fusion over implicated segments if deemed suitable candidate for surgery:
  - If poor surgical candidate with poor life expectancy, medical management recommended
  - Surgery may be done anteriorly, posteriorly, or combined two-stage approach for added stabilization
  - May include a combination of the following techniques: Laminectomy (entire lamina, thickened ligaments, and part of enlarged facet joints removed to relieve pressure), Laminotomy (section of lamina and ligament removed), Foraminotomy (expanding space of neural foramen by removing soft tissues, small disk fragments, and bony spurs in the locus), Laminoplasty (expanding space within spinal canal by repositioning lamina), Diskectomy (removal of section of herniated disk), Corpectomy (removal of vertebral body and disks), Bony Spur Removal
  - Thoracic Decompression/Fusion Approaches
- Anterior transthoracic (see ▶ Fig. 2.18):
  - Excellent exposure to anterior thoracic spine, vertebral bodies, intervertebral disks, spinal canal, and nerve roots
  - Posterior elements and contralateral pedicle inaccessible
  - No extensive bone resection or corpectomy
  - Can freely use hemostatic agents in locus of bone removal since lateral fusion is performed
  - Do not perform if there is displacement of posterior bone elements into spinal canal or when posterior penetrating injury exists (unless as part of a combined procedure)
  - T2–T9 is preferentially approached from the right side to avoid injury to heart, aortic arch, and great vessels
  - T10–L2 is preferentially approached from the left side to avoid injury to liver

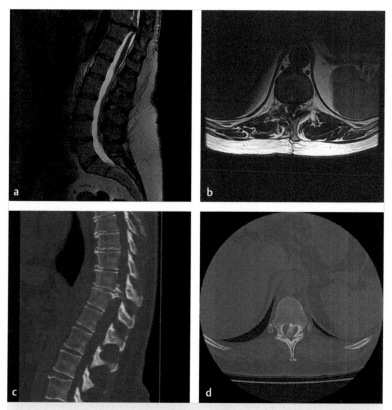

**Fig. 2.18 (a–d)** A middle-aged woman with a calcified T10–T11 thoracic protrusion previously failed to be removed via a posterior posterolateral approach. A right anterior transthoracic decompression and reconstruction were employed instead. Preoperative images reveal calcification of T10/T11 herniation.

- Anterior transsternal (see ▶ Fig. 2.19):
  - Direct anterior exposure of thoracic spine
  - Excellent for upper thoracic access and cervicothoracic exposure

## Indications for Surgical Intervention

- Spinal stenosis
- No sufficient improvement of pain and other symptoms after nonoperative measures (physical therapy, medications/injections, pain management)

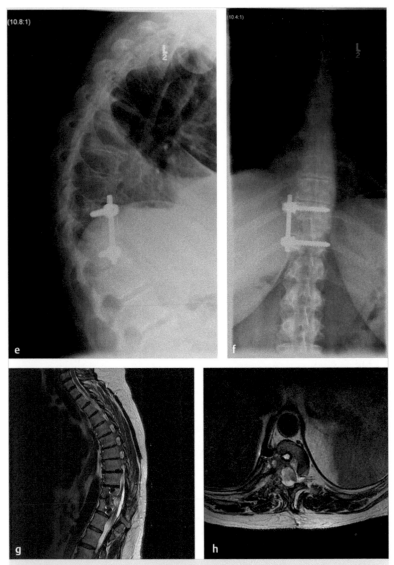

**Fig. 2.18** (*Continued*) **(e–h)** Follow-up images (12 months) demonstrating fusion instrumentation and thoracic decompression. The patient's preoperative axial and lower limb pain was resolved through the transthoracic approach. (Source: Transthoracic diskectomy: anterior approach . In: Nader R, Berta S, Gragnanielllo C, et al, eds. Neurosurgery Tricks of the Trade: Spine and Peripheral Nerves. 1st ed. Thieme; 2014).

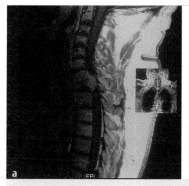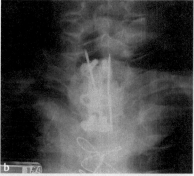

**Fig. 2.19** A middle-aged man with an invasive tumor that damaged the T1 vertebral body (**a**) received thoracic decompression and reconstruction via a transsternal approach. Instrumentation ensured stabilization (**b**). (Source: Operative technique. In: Dickman C, Fehlings M, Gokaslan Z, eds. Spinal Cord and Spinal Column Tumors. 1st ed. Thieme; 2006).

- Spinal condition isolated to specific locus of the body
- Significant reduction in everyday activities due to symptoms
- Expected postsurgical favorable outcome
- Partial paraplegia
- Residual thoracic compression
- Existence of blunt chest trauma or potential hemorrhagic lesions
- Sufficient disruption of supporting ligaments
- Transthoracic/Transsternal Approaches:
  - Partial injury of thoracic cord
  - Anterior compression
  - No intraspinal displacement of posterior bone elements
  - Anterior spinal cord syndrome with partial or complete myelographic spinal block
  - Thoracic disk disease
  - Vertebral osteomyelitis of diskitis

## Surgical Procedure for Anterior Transthoracic Decompression/Fusion

1. Informed consent signed, preoperative labs normal, no Aspirin/Plavix/Coumadin/NSAIDs/Celebrex/Naprosyn/other anticoagulants and anti-inflammatory drugs for at least 2 weeks
2. Appropriate intubation and sedation and lines (if necessary) as per the anesthetist

3. Large bore (16–14 gauge) IV access for blood loss during operation
4. Patient placed in left/right lateral decubitus position with all pressure points padded (depending on whether left or right lateral thoracotomy will be performed)
5. Neuromonitoring may be required to monitor nerves (if necessary and indicated)
6. Intraoperative fluoroscopy used as deemed appropriate
7. Time out is performed with agreement from everyone in the room for correct patient and correct surgery with consent signed
8. Make posterior incision starting from appropriate level of spine, curving down the line of the rib
9. Divide the latissimus and trapezius muscles:
   a. Divide the rhomboids and both teres as well for T1–T4 exposure
10. Mobilize scapula from chest wall and elevate using scapula retractor
11. Enter chest through intercostal space or the bed of the rib at the level of vertebrae of interest:
    a. Make incision in intercostal space to enter thoracic cavity
    b. Resect proximal rib as bone graft will be used
    c. Mobilize erector spinae superiorly and inferiorly, or divide it transversely at the level of intercostal incision
    d. Retract ribs and scapula using Finochietto or Burford retractor
    e. Retract the intercostal space
12. Expose the vertebrae of interest:
    a. Mobilize superior and posterior hilum (T1–T4)
    b. Mobilize the pulmonary ligament and hilar pleura
    c. Divide the mediastinal pleura posterior to the hilum from the inferior pulmonary vein to just above the mainstem bronchus (T5–T8)
    d. Displace the lung anteriorly and move it out of the way using wet lap pads
    e. Open the mediastinal pleura anterior to the vertebral bodies vertically from the thoracic inlet to the level of the carina. Dissect and mobilize the mediastinal structures. Mobilize the azygos vein with tributaries and the esophagus using blunt and sharp dissection (right thoracotomy), or mobilize the descending thoracic aorta (left thoracotomy) (T1–T8)
    f. Mobilize the thoracic duct anteriorly (T5–T8)
    g. Retract diaphragm using sponge stick. Mobilize posterior attachments of diaphragm. Mobilize posterior mediastinal structures for anterior retraction (T9–T12)
13. Perform the decompression procedure over the desired segments based on preoperative imaging of levels that are compressed due to trauma:
    a. Using Leksell rongeurs and hand-held high-speed air drill, resect the adjacent disk material immediately ventral to the posterior cortical bone of the vertebral bodies

    b. Leave a thin shelf of bone immediately adjacent to posterior longitudinal ligament and dura intact

    c. A complete corpectomy (removal of entire vertebral body) may be needed in certain cases to decompress the spinal cord:

        i. This step avoids the cord falling ventrally, which can result in cord injury during the resection process

    d. Remove adequate portion of subcortical bone, using high-speed air drill, across midline for decompression of ventral cord surface

    e. Remove thin shelf of bone adjacent to posterior longitudinal ligament with rongeur

    f. Control bone bleeding with bone wax

14. Perform posterior thoracic fusion with instrumentation with patient in prone position (may not be needed):

    a. Place and secure bone graft with cancellous screws to bridge the vertebra above and below the midpoint of the fracture, avoiding injury to vital structures

15. Achieve hemostasis
16. Drain the chest and inspect posterior mediastinum for lymph leak
17. If previously mobilized, reattach the diaphragm to the fascia of the posterior chest wall with sutures
18. Close the muscle and skin incisions in appropriate fashion, often with placement of postoperative chest tube that can be removed after 2 to 3 days

## Surgical Procedure for Anterior Transsternal Decompression/Fusion

1. Informed consent signed, preoperative labs normal, no Aspirin/Plavix/Coumadin/NSAIDs/Celebrex/Naprosyn/other anticoagulants and anti-inflammatory drugs for at least 2 weeks
2. Appropriate intubation and sedation and lines (if necessary) as per the anesthetist
3. Patient placed in supine position with all pressure points padded
4. Neuromonitoring may be required to monitor nerves (if necessary and indicated)
5. Time out is performed with agreement from everyone in the room for correct patient and correct surgery with consent signed
6. Make an incision on medial border of right sternocleidomastoid, extending down over manubrium
7. Perform median sternotomy with sternal saw
8. Mobilize sternocleidomastoid laterally and trachea/esophagus medially, exposing anterior cervicothoracic spine

9. Perform the decompression procedure over the desired segments based on preoperative imaging of levels that are compressed due to trauma:
   a. Using Leksell rongeurs and hand-held high-speed drill, perform a corpectomy or diskectomy to decompress the spinal cord
   b. Place cage and anterior plate
10. Perform spinal fusion with instrumentation posteriorly with patient flipped to prone position if needed:
    a. Perform reconstruction with expandable cage and autograft
    b. Perform screw-plate fixation
11. After appropriate hemostasis is obtained, muscle and skin incisions can then be closed in appropriate fashion, often with placement of postoperative Jackson-Pratt drains:
    a. Achieve closure of sternum with sternal wires

## Pitfalls

- Reduction in range of motion and mobility of fused spinal segments
- Intraoperative CSF leak
- Blood clot (deep vein thrombosis, or more severe pulmonary embolism)
- Damage to spinal nerves and/or cord
- Postoperative weakness or numbness or continued pain
- Postoperative wound infection
- Continued symptoms postsurgically/unresolved symptoms with no improvement to quality of life
- Prolonged hospitalization due to invasiveness of surgery and other comorbidities/iatrogenic infection
- Loss of sensation
- Progressive kyphosis
- Residual spinal compression
- Problems with bowel/bladder control
- Injury to artery of Adamkiewicz (generally originating from the left T8–L1) resulting in cord ischemia, radicular arteries (typically accomplished during dissection around intervertebral foramina), thoracic duct, chylothorax, and/or esophagus (from transthoracic approach)
- Vascular complications
- Atelectasis and pneumonia
- Hemothorax and empyema (managed with drainage and antibiotics)
- Injury to carotid sheath, trachea, esophagus, recurrent laryngeal nerves, great vessels, vertebral arteries, and/or sympathetic trunk (from transsternal approach)

## Prognosis

- Hospitalization rates depend on the type of procedure performed, preoperative examination status, and patient's age/comorbidities
- Pain medications for postsurgical pain
- After fusion, halt use of all NSAIDs for 6 months
- Catheter placed in bladder and removed 1 to 2 days after surgery
- Physical therapy and occupational therapy will be needed postoperatively as outpatient to regain strength
- Brace (i.e., Jewett or Taylor type) placed after discharge (patient can be mobilized after 2 to 3 weeks of transthoracic decompression/fusion operation)

# 2.3 Tumor/Vascular

## 2.3.1 Anterior and Posterior Approaches for Thoracic Tumor Resection (Vertebral Pathology)

### Symptoms and Signs

- Incidental with symptoms (depending on size and location)
- Paraplegia (partial or complete)
- Diminished control of bowel/bladder function
- Moderate/severe back pain
- Difficulty maintaining balance and walking
- Loss of sensation in hands
- Inability to conduct fine motor skills with hands

### Surgical Pathology

- Thoracic spine benign/malignant tumor

### Diagnostic Modalities

- CT of thoracic spine with and without contrast to assess whether there is bony involvement of tumor
- MRI of thoracic spine with and without contrast to assess if there is spinal cord, epidural space or nerve root involvement of tumor
- PET scan of body to look for other foci of tumor
- CT of chest/abdomen/pelvis to rule out metastatic disease

## Differential Diagnosis

- Metastatic tumor
  - Breast, prostate, lung, renal cell
- Primary tumor
  - Schwannoma, neurofibroma, myeloma, plasmacytoma, meningioma, ependymoma, astrocytoma, hemangioblastoma, lipoma, dermoid, epidermoid, teratoma, neuroblastoma, oligodendroglioma, cholesteatoma, subependymoma, osteosarcoma, chondrosarcoma, Ewing's sarcoma, chordoma, lymphoma, osteoid osteoma, aneurysmal bone cyst, eosinophilic granuloma, angiolipoma

## Treatment Options

- Acute pain control with medications and pain management
- If asymptomatic or mildly symptomatic with neck pain/radiculopathy with small focus of tumor:
  - Radiation treatment (radiation oncology consultation)
  - Some metastatic tumors are radioresistant
  - Chemotherapy (medical oncology consultation)
  - Some metastatic tumors are radioresistant
  - Kyphoplasty (to treat pain)
  - Surgical instrumentation and fusion (if there is concern for deformity, instability, or cord compression)
- If symptomatic with cord compression and myelopathy with large tumor burden:
  - Urgent surgical decompression and fusion over multiple segments with tumor resection if deemed suitable candidate for surgery; may be followed by radiation treatment after resection if considered necessary by the radiation oncologist:
  - Oncologist will need to determine overall prognosis, Karnofsky performance score, and extent of visceral disease
  - If poor surgical candidate with poor life expectancy, medical management recommended
  - Surgery may be done anteriorly, posteriorly, or combined two-stage approach for added stabilization
  - Preoperative embolization may be indicated for select vascular tumors to the spine such as renal cell cancer, thyroid cancer, breast cancer, etc. in order to decrease vascularity intraoperatively

## Indications for Surgical Intervention

- Spinal stenosis

- No improvement after nonoperative therapy (physical therapy, pain management)
- Paraplegia
- Cord compression with or without myelopathy
- To obtain diagnosis if no other site for biopsy is available
- Risk of pathological fractures without stabilization

## Surgical Procedure for Posterior Thoracic Spine

1. Informed consent signed, preoperative labs normal, no Aspirin/Plavix/ Coumadin/NSAIDs/Celebrex/Naprosyn/other anticoagulants and anti-inflammatory drugs for at least 2 weeks
2. Appropriate intubation and sedation and lines (if necessary) as per the anesthetist
3. Patient placed prone on Jackson Table with all pressure points padded
4. Neuromonitoring may be required to monitor nerves
5. Time out is performed with agreement from everyone in the room for correct patient and correct surgery with consent signed
6. Make an incision down the midline of back, over the vertebrae where laminectomy is to be performed
7. Perform subperiosteal dissection of muscles bilaterally exposing the spinous process and paraspinal muscles
8. Dissect tissue planes along spinous process and laminae using rongeurs
9. Move paraspinal muscles laterally to expose the laminae
10. Once the locus of interest is exposed, it is best to localize and verify the correct vertebrae via X-ray or fluoroscopic imaging and confirming with at least two people in the room
11. Perform the laminectomy over the desired segments based on preoperative imaging of levels that are compressed due to tumor:
    a. Using Leksell rongeurs and hand-held high-speed drill, remove the bony spinous process and bilateral lamina as indicated for specific procedure
    b. Remove the thick ligamentum flavum with Kerrison rongeurs with careful dissection beneath the ligament to ensure no adhesions exist to dura mater below and thus avoiding CSF leak
    c. Perform appropriate foraminotomy with Kerrison rongeurs as needed for appropriate decompression of nerve roots
    d. Identify location of tumor and resect tumor as needed if within the lamina, epidural, or within the spinal canal/cord (see ▶ Fig. 2.20):
       i. If within the lamina or epidural in nature, the tumor can be visualized immediately and removed gently
       ii. If within the spinal cord, use operative microscope and open the spinal cord dura midline with 11 blade and tack up the dural leaflets with suture

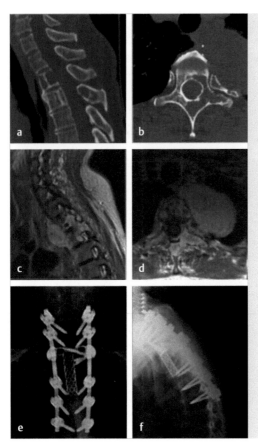

**Fig. 2.20** A middle-aged woman with a capillary hemangioma, associated with the thoracic apex and extending into T2–T3 (**a–d**), received a posterolateral corpectomy (T2–T3) and fusion with posterior instrumentation of C7–T6 (**e, f**). The success of the cervicothoracic corpectomy was verified via postoperative X-ray. (Source: Cervicothoracic corpectomy. In: Fessler R, Sekhar L, eds. Atlas of Neurosurgical Techniques: Spine and Peripheral Nerves. 2nd ed. Thieme; 2016).

   iii. If tumor is intradural and extramedullary, the tumor can then be resected carefully with microdissection technique without cord injury (neuromonitoring needed in these cases)

   iv. If tumor is intradural and intramedullary, with microdissection technique the cord must be entered midline and the tumor must be identified and resected starting centrally first, then around the edges (neuromonitoring needed in these cases)

12. After appropriate tumor resection, there may be need for additional stabilization to prevent kyphosis if the resection caused multiple segment decompression. Therefore, instrumentation with lateral mass screws can be placed over segments involved with rods bilaterally and fusion/arthrodesis along these segments (see ▶ Fig. 2.21 and ▶ Fig. 2.22).

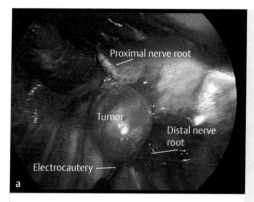

**Fig. 2.21** Intraoperative image (a) and illustration (b) of thoracoscopic-assisted tumor resection (not involving foramen). (Source: Thoracoscopic resection of paraspinal tumors. In: Nader R, Berta S, Gragnanielllo C, et al, eds. Neurosurgery Tricks of the Trade: Spine and Peripheral Nerves. 1st ed. Thieme; 2014).

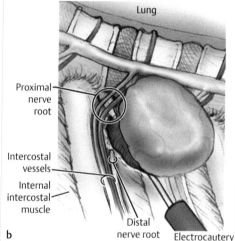

13. After appropriate hemostasis is obtained, muscle and skin incisions can then be closed in appropriate fashion, often with placement of postoperative drains that can be removed after 2 to 3 days.

## Surgical Procedure for Anterior Thoracic Spine

1. Informed consent signed, preoperative labs normal, no Aspirin/Plavix/Coumadin/NSAIDs/Celebrex/Naprosyn/other anticoagulants and anti-inflammatory drugs for at least 2 weeks
2. Appropriate intubation and sedation and lines (if necessary) as per the anesthetist

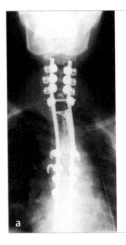 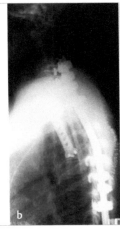

**Fig. 2.22** (a, b) Postoperative radiographs of a patient who had a left superior sulcus tumor. The patient received a laminectomy (T1–T3), a vertebrectomy (T1 and T2), and fusion with instrumentation. (Source: Management options. In: Dickman C, Fehlings M, Gokaslan Z, eds. Spinal Cord and Spinal Column Tumors. 1st ed. Thieme; 2006).

3. Patient placed in supine position, breathing through endotracheal tube with ventilator, with transverse shoulder roll if C7–T2 is indicated
4. Neuromonitoring may be required to monitor nerves (if necessary and indicated)
5. Time out is performed with agreement from everyone in the room for correct patient and correct surgery with consent signed
6. Initial operation actions depend on the approach:
   a. Cervicothoracic approach (C7–T2):
      i. Perform oblique incision anterior to sternocleidomastoid muscle
      ii. Retract sternocleidomastoid muscle and carotid sheath laterally
      iii. Retract laryngeal mechanism, thyroid, and esophagus medially
      iv. Place Finochietto retractor and perform a manubrial split
      v. Insert nasogastric tube to identify cervical esophagus
      vi. Enter prevertebral space, exposing lower cervical and upper thoracic (a Weitlaner retractor can be inserted to enhance exposure)
   b. T3–T10 approach (typically followed for thoracotomy):
      i. Enter chest two interspaces above the vertebrae of interest
      ii. Resect rib below incision (can be used in autograft if necessary)
      iii. Notch adjacent inferior rib to increase exposure
      iv. Utilize Bookwalter retraction system to retract chest wall, lung, and diaphragm
      v. Maintain rib separation with two shallow bladder blades and maintain downward traction on lung and diaphragm using deep straight blades

   c. Thoracoabdominal approach (T11–L2):
      i. Resect the tenth rib and divide the ipsilateral hemidiaphragm circumferentially
      ii. Utilize Bookwalter retraction system to retract peritoneal contents and liver
      iii. Mobilize psoas musculature to access the vertebrae of interest

7. Once the vertebrae of interest are exposed, it is best to localize and verify the correct vertebrae via X-ray or fluoroscopic imaging and confirming with at least two people in the room

8. Perform the laminectomy over the desired segments based on preoperative imaging of levels that are compressed due to tumor:
   a. Using Leksell rongeurs and hand-held high-speed drill, remove the bony spinous process and bilateral lamina as indicated for specific procedure
   b. Remove the thick ligamentum flavum with Kerrison rongeurs with careful dissection beneath the ligament to ensure no adhesions exist to dura mater below and thus avoiding CSF leak
   c. Perform appropriate foraminotomy with Kerrison rongeurs as needed for appropriate decompression of nerve roots
   d. Identify location of tumor and resect tumor as needed if within the lamina, epidural, or within the spinal canal/cord (with care not to injure the vertebral artery)
      i. If within the lamina or epidural in nature, the tumor can be visualized immediately and removed gently
      ii. If within the spinal cord, use operative microscope and open the spinal cord dura midline with 11 blade and tack up the dural leaflets with suture
      iii. If tumor is intradural and extramedullary, the tumor can then be resected carefully with microdissection technique without cord injury (neuromonitoring needed in these cases)
      iv. If tumor is intradural and intramedullary, with microdissection technique the cord must be entered midline and the tumor must be identified and resected starting centrally first, then around the edges (neuromonitoring needed in these cases)

9. Place chest tube if significant pleural tear occurs (can be removed in 2–3 days)

10. After appropriate tumor resection, there may be need for additional stabilization to prevent kyphosis if the resection caused multiple segment decompression. Therefore, instrumentation with lateral mass screws can be placed over segments involved with rods bilaterally and fusion/arthrodesis along these segments.

11. After appropriate hemostasis is obtained, muscle and skin incisions can then be closed in appropriate fashion, often with placement of postoperative Jackson-Pratt drains that can be removed after 2 to 3 days

## Pitfalls

- Reduction in range of motion and mobility of fused spinal segments if fusion is performed
- Intraoperative CSF leak
- Blood clot (deep vein thrombosis, or more severe pulmonary embolism)
- Damage to spinal nerves and/or cord
- Postoperative weakness or numbness or continued pain
- Postoperative wound infection
- Continued symptoms postsurgically/unresolved symptoms with no improvement to quality of life
- Prolonged hospitalization due to invasiveness of surgery and other comorbidities/iatrogenic infection
- Progressive kyphosis
- Residual spinal compression
- Problems with bowel/bladder control

## Prognosis

- Hospitalization rates depend on the type of procedure performed, preoperative examination status, and patient's age/comorbidities
- Pain medications for postsurgical pain
- Physical therapy and occupational therapy will be needed postoperatively, immediately and as outpatient to regain strength
- Catheter placed in bladder and removed 1 to 2 days after surgery
- Brace placed after discharge to immobilize to increase rate of healing

## 2.3.2 Thoracic Anterior and Posterior Approaches for Vascular Lesion Resection (Vertebral Pathology)

### Symptoms and Signs

- Dilated arteries and veins with dysplastic vessels
- Subarachnoid hemorrhage
- Myelopathy
- Seizure
- Ischemic injury to thoracic spine
- Increased sweating around thoracic vascular lesion

- Paraplegia (partial or complete)
- Diminished control of bowel/bladder function
- Moderate/severe back pain
- Difficulty maintaining balance and walking
- Loss of sensation in hands
- Inability to conduct fine motor skills in hands
- Paresis/paralysis
- Hemorrhaging

## Surgical Pathology

- Thoracic vascular benign/malignant lesions

## Diagnostic Modalities

- Angiography
  - Preoperative spinal angiography
  - Intraoperative indocyanine green (ICG) angiography
- CT of thoracic spine with and without contrast (can rule out acute hemorrhage)
- MRI of thoracic spine with and without contrast

## Differential Diagnosis FMD

- Spinal AVM (see ▶ Fig. 2.23)
  - Intradural-intramedullary (hemorrhaging common)
    i. Glomus (Type II)
    ○ Juvenile (Type III)
  - Intradural-extramedullary
  - Conus medullaris
  - Metameric
  - Extradural
  - Cavernoma
  - Capillary telangiectasia
- Spinal dural AVF (Type I) (see ▶ Fig. 2.24)
  - Intradural-extramedullary
    ii. Perimedullary AVF (Type IV)
  - Intradural-intramedullary
  - Extradural
- Vertebral sarcoidosis
- Dissection syndromes

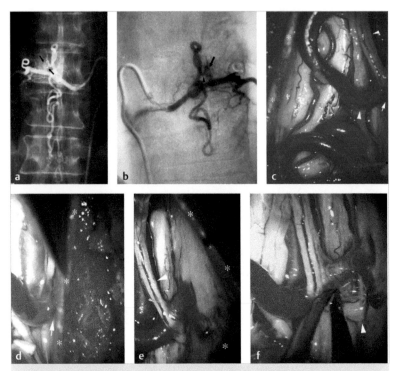

**Fig. 2.23** A dural arteriovenous fistula (AVF) was found in the right T9 nerve root; *arrows* point to the nidus (**a, b**). The dura was resected to visualize the nerve root and the arterialized medullary vein draining blood from the AVF (**c–f**). (Source: Operative procedure. In: Macdonald R, ed. Neurosurgical Operative Atlas: Vascular Neurosurgery. 3rd ed. Thieme; 2018).

## Treatment Options

- Conservative observation
- Radiation treatment
  - Conventional radiation (not very effective therapy)
  - Stereotactic radiosurgery and radiotherapy (nidus must not be greater than 3 cm in diameter)
- Surgery
  - Microsurgical resection
  - Preferred option if bleeding or seizures result from lesion

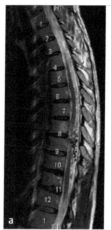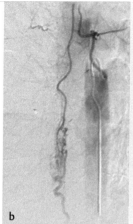

**Fig. 2.24** MRI scan reveals vascular flow voids at T8–T9, suggesting an arteriovenous malformation (AVM) (**a**). A thoracic angiography confirms the AVM (**b**). (Source: Spinal arteriovenous fistulas and malformations. In: Nader R, Berta S, Gragnaniello C, et al, eds. Neurosurgery Tricks of the Trade: Spine and Peripheral Nerves. 1st ed. Thieme; 2014).

- Endovascular embolization using the following embolic agents (initial procedure to facilitate surgery):
  - Coils: Close down vessel supplying AVM (cannot independently treat AVM nidus)
  - Onyx: Solidifies, forming a cast, in vessel supplying AVM (best penetration of AVM nidus)
  - N-butyl cyanoacrylate (tissue adhesive): Solidifies as a glue in vessel supplying AVM (greater risks and worse outcomes than with Onyx)
  - Polyvinyl alcohol: Used prior to craniotomy or surgical resection of AVM (cannot independently treat AVM pathology)
- Combination techniques
  - Embolization followed by stereotactic radiosurgery
- Venous angiomas should not be treated unless certainly contributing to intractable seizures and bleeding

## Indications for Endovascular Intervention

- Preoperative embolization (for surgical AVM resection)
- Presence of associated lesions (aneurysms/pseudoaneurysms on feeding pedicle or nidus, venous thrombosis, venous outflow restriction, venous pouches, dilatations)
- Small surgically inaccessible AVM treated by curative AVM embolization or radiosurgery

- Palliative treatment when symptomatic AVM not entirely treatable by the other approaches
- Paraplegia
- Cord compression with or without myelopathy

## Surgical Procedure for Thoracic Spine (Laminoplasty; Preferred over Laminectomy Due to Increased Preservation of Neural Structures)

1. Administer 20 mg propranolol orally four times a day for 3 days to patient preoperation
2. Informed consent signed, preoperative labs normal, no Aspirin/Plavix/Coumadin/NSAIDs/Celebrex/Naprosyn/other anticoagulants and anti-inflammatory drugs for at least 2 weeks
3. Administer preoperative prophylactic IV antibiotics
4. Appropriate intubation and sedation and lines (if considered necessary as per the anesthetist)
5. Patient placed prone on gel rolls, pressure points padded
6. Neuromonitoring may be required to monitor nerves
7. Time out is performed with agreement from everyone in the room for correct patient and correct surgery with consent signed
8. C-arm fluoroscopy equipment set up in operation zone
9. Make an incision over the vertebrae where laminoplasty is to be performed:
   a. Prepare to utilize one level above and below the AVM nidus or AVF shunt
   b. Extension to ipsilateral pedicle performed if deemed necessary to enhance lateral of the AVM nidus or AVF shunt
10. Perform subperiosteal dissection of muscles bilaterally to expose the vertebra
11. Once the bone is exposed, it is best to localize and verify the correct vertebra via X-ray or fluoroscopic imaging and confirming with at least two people in the room
12. Bovie electrocautery is used to progress dissection toward the spine and to attain hemostasis, with the help of bipolar forceps
13. Move musculature around vertebra laterally and downward to expose the dura
14. Utilize self-retaining retractors to keep everything in place
15. Open the dura, followed by the arachnoid
16. Clip the arachnoid to the dural edges using self-retaining retractors to reveal the vascular lesion source

17. Video-angiography (typically with ICG) is used to visualize the blood flow through the AVM
18. If the AVM nidus is intraparenchymal in its entirety, prepare to perform a myelotomy (midline dorsal, dorsal root entry zone, lateral, and anterior midline types). Otherwise, continue with the laminoplasty procedure (typically a pial resection).
19. Using the surgical suction and nonstick bipolar forceps, the pia arachnoid is revealed
20. Cut and coagulate the appropriate vessels
21. Separate AVM from the spinal cord using surgical scissors, bipolar, and suction
22. Several nerve rootlets will be tangled with the AVM (they may be tangled with dorsal nerve roots) and must be removed by necessity, others may be left unaltered
23. Cut the dentate ligament where it is attached to the AVM
24. The spinal canal is further exposed, revealing the feeders of the AVM
25. Use ICG video-angiography to confirm no further shunting of the arterial venous blood
26. Close the dura as well as the subcutaneous tissues after the laminoplasty is successfully performed
27. Close the skin with suture, skin-glue, steri-strips, or surgical staples
28. Postoperative injection of the relevant artery and vertebral locus demonstrate that the AVM has been treated

## Surgical Procedure for Thoracic Spine (Laminectomy)

1. Follow laminoplasty procedure above until initial hemostasis is completed and self-retaining retractors are placed, keeping the musculature set aside
2. Use Leksell rongeurs and high-speed burr drill to remove the posterior spinous processes and bilateral lamina
3. Remove the free ligamentum flavum using Kerrison rongeurs to decompress the nerve roots
4. Open the lamina via "green-stick" fracture technique
5. Utilizing Adson Periosteal Elevator, elevate lamina from the side (do not slide underneath it)
6. Fasten plates and screws at the lateral borders of each lamina and the facet joint, stabilizing the spine if deformity or instability is noted
7. Wash the wound with antibiotic saline solution and re-achieve hemostasis via Bovie electrocautery and bipolar, applying local anesthetic to the wound to reduce bleeding

8. Place a postoperative drain (can be removed after 2–3 days)
9. Close the fascia and subcutaneous tissue with Vicryl
10. Close the skin with suture, skin-glue, steri-strips, or surgical staples

## Embolization Procedure (Onyx)

1. Shake Onyx vial on mixer for 20 minutes. Onyx-18 is common, Onyx-34 is suitable for very high flow AVMs, and Onyx-500 is used in aneurysm embolization treatments
2. Wedge microcatheter tip into arterial branch supplying the AVM, preferably very close to the AVM nidus
3. Perform angiography through the microcatheter to confirm that the arterial branch exclusively supplies the AVM
4. Prime the DMSO-compatible microcatheter (marathon, echelon, rebar, ultraflow) with 0.3 to 0.8 mL DMSO so that Onyx does not solidify in the microcatheter
5. Slowly inject Onyx solution, allowing no more than 1 cm of reflux. If reflux occurs, continue after 1 to 2 minute waiting period
6. Halt injection when Onyx no longer flows into the nidus, but refluxes instead

## Pitfalls

- Stroke
- Intraoperative and postoperative bleeding
- Failure to remove entire vascular lesion source
- Future recurrence of vascular lesion
- Recompression of thoracic spinal cord
- Postlaminoplasty kyphosis
- Nerve root palsies
- Damage to spinal nerves and/or cord
- Postoperative weakness or numbness or continued pain
- Postoperative wound infection
- Prolonged hospitalization due to invasiveness of surgery and other comorbidities/iatrogenic infection
- Temporary postoperative paresthesia
- Iatrogenic vertebral artery injury during embolization process

## Prognosis (AVM Laminoplasty)

- Admit patient to intensive care unit (ICU)
- Keep leg on the side used during procedure straight for 2 hours (if angioseal closure) or 6 to 8 hours (if manual compression), keeping head of bed elevated 15 degrees

- Check groins, distal pulse (DP')s, vitals, and neuro checks q 15 min ×4, q 30 min ×4, then q hr
- Maintain mild hypotension for 12 to 72 hours post-op
- Monitor patient for perfusion pressure break through bleeding, seizures, and other possible complications
- Review/resume preprocedure medications (hold metformin 48 hours postprocedure; continue oral hypoglycemics until satisfactory oral intake)
- Schedule outpatient appointment 4 weeks postprocedure
- Angiography (not computed tomography angiography [CTA] or magnetic resonance angiography [MRA]) 1 and 5 years postprocedure (AVM), or MRI 3 months postprocedure, depending on the cause of lesion (spinal cavernous malformations)

## Prognosis (AVM Laminectomy)

- Hospitalization rates depend on the type of procedure performed, preoperative examination status, and patient's age/comorbidities
- Physical therapy and occupational therapy will be needed postoperatively, immediately and as outpatient to regain strength
- Brace will be used for 8 weeks after discharge to immobilize to increase rate of healing

## 2.3.3 Thoracic Anterior and Posterior Techniques for Tumor Resection (Spinal Canal Pathology)

### Symptoms and Signs

- Incidental with symptoms (depending on size and location)
- Paraplegia (partial or complete)
- Diminished control of bowel/bladder function
- Moderate/severe back pain
- Difficulty maintaining balance and walking
- Loss of sensation in hands
- Inability to conduct fine motor skills with hands

### Surgical Pathology

- Thoracic spine benign/malignant tumor

### Diagnostic Modalities

- CT of thoracic spine with and without contrast to assess whether there is bony involvement of tumor

- MRI of thoracic spine with and without contrast to assess if there is spinal cord, epidural space, or nerve root involvement of tumor
- PET scan of body to look for other foci of tumor
- CT of chest/abdomen/pelvis to rule out metastatic disease
- X-ray (not as reliable for tumor diagnosis)
- Biopsy to examine tissue sample to determine whether tumor is benign or malignant, and what cancer type resulted in the tumor if malignancy is determined

## Differential Diagnosis

- Metastatic tumor
  - Breast, prostate, lung, renal cell
- Primary tumor
  - Schwannoma, neurofibroma, myeloma, plasmacytoma, meningioma, ependymoma, astrocytoma, hemangioblastoma, lipoma, dermoid, epidermoid, teratoma, neuroblastoma, oligodendroglioma, cholesteatoma, subependymoma, osteosarcoma, chondrosarcoma, Ewing's sarcoma, chordoma, lymphoma, osteoid osteoma, aneurysmal bone cyst, eosinophilic granuloma, angiolipoma

## Treatment Options

- If asymptomatic or mildly symptomatic with neck pain/radiculopathy with small focus of tumor:
  - Radiation treatment (radiation oncology consultation)
  - Some metastatic tumors are radioresistant
  - Chemotherapy (medical oncology consultation)
  - Some metastatic tumors are radioresistant
  - Kyphoplasty (to treat pain)
  - Surgical instrumentation and fusion (if there is concern for deformity, instability, or cord compression)
- If symptomatic with cord compression and myelopathy with large tumor burden:
  - Urgent surgical decompression and fusion over multiple segments with tumor resection if deemed suitable candidate for surgery; may be followed by radiation treatment after resection if considered necessary by the radiation oncologist
  - Oncologist will need to determine overall prognosis, Karnofsky performance score, and extent of visceral disease
  - If poor surgical candidate with poor life expectancy, medical management recommended

- Surgery may be done anteriorly, posteriorly, or combined two-stage approach for added stabilization
- Preoperative embolization may be indicated for select vascular tumors to the spine such as renal cell cancer, thyroid cancer, breast cancer, etc. in order to decrease vascularity intraoperatively

## Indications for Surgical Intervention

- Spinal stenosis
- No improvement after nonoperative therapy (physical therapy, pain management)
- Paraplegia
- Cord compression with or without myelopathy
- To obtain diagnosis if no other site for biopsy is available
- Risk of pathological fractures without stabilization

## Surgical Procedure for Posterior Thoracic Spine

1. Informed consent signed, preoperative labs normal, no Aspirin/Plavix/Coumadin/NSAIDs/Celebrex/Naprosyn/other anticoagulants and anti-inflammatory drugs for at least 2 weeks
2. Appropriate intubation and sedation and lines (if necessary) as per the anesthetist
3. Patient placed prone in neutral alignment on Jackson Table with all pressure points padded
4. Neuromonitoring may be required to monitor nerves
5. Time out is performed with agreement from everyone in the room for correct patient and correct surgery with consent signed
6. Make an incision down the midline of back, over the vertebrae where laminectomy is to be performed
7. Perform subperiosteal dissection of muscles bilaterally to expose the spinous process and paraspinal muscles
8. Dissect tissue planes along spinous process and laminae using rongeurs
9. Move paraspinal muscles laterally to expose the laminae
10. Once the locus of interest is exposed, it is best to localize and verify the correct vertebrae via X-ray or fluoroscopic imaging and confirming with at least two people in the room
11. Perform the laminectomy over the desired segments based on preoperative imaging of levels that are compressed due to tumor:
    a. Using Leksell rongeurs and hand-held high-speed drill, remove the bony spinous process and bilateral lamina as indicated for specific procedure

b. Remove the thick ligamentum flavum with Kerrison rongeurs with careful dissection beneath the ligament to ensure no adhesions exist to dura mater below and thus avoiding CSF leak

c. Perform appropriate foraminotomy with Kerrison rongeurs as needed for appropriate decompression of nerve roots

d. Identify location of tumor and resect tumor as needed within the spinal canal

    i. Use operative microscope and open the spinal cord dura midline with 11 blade and tack up the dural leaflets with suture

    ii. If tumor is intradural and extramedullary, the tumor can then be resected carefully with microdissection technique without cord injury (neuromonitoring needed in these cases)

    iii. If tumor is intradural and intramedullary, with microdissection technique the cord must be entered midline and the tumor must be identified and resected starting centrally first, then around the edges (neuromonitoring needed in these cases)

12. After appropriate tumor resection, there may be need for additional stabilization to prevent kyphosis if the resection caused multiple segment decompression. Therefore, instrumentation with pedicle screws can be placed over segments involved with rods bilaterally and fusion/arthrodesis along these segments (see ▶ Fig. 2.25)

13. After appropriate hemostasis is obtained, muscle and skin incisions can then be closed in appropriate fashion, often with placement of postoperative drains that can be removed after 2 to 3 days

## Surgical Procedure for Anterior Thoracic Spine

1. Informed consent signed, preoperative labs normal, no Aspirin/Plavix/Coumadin/NSAIDs/Celebrex/Naprosyn/other anticoagulants and anti-inflammatory drugs for at least 2 weeks

2. Appropriate intubation and sedation and lines (if necessary) as per the anesthetist

3. Patient placed in supine position, breathing through endotracheal tube with ventilator, with transverse shoulder roll if C7–T2 is indicated

4. Neuromonitoring may be required to monitor nerves (if necessary and indicated)

5. Time out is performed with agreement from everyone in the room for correct patient and correct surgery with consent signed

6. Initial operation actions depend on the approach:

    a. Cervicothoracic approach (C7–T2):

        i. Perform oblique incision anterior to sternocleidomastoid muscle

        ii. Retract sternocleidomastoid muscle and carotid sheath laterally

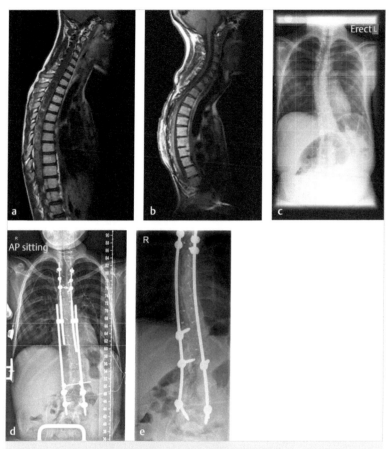

**Fig. 2.25** MRI scan reveals intradural thoracic glioma (**a**). Resection, radiotherapy, and chemotherapy were performed, removing the tumor but resulting in thoracic kyphosis and scoliosis (**b, c**). Instrumentation (growing dual rods) was added to allow for growth (**d**), later to be replaced by fusion and instrumentation for stabilization (**e**). (Source: Intradural tumors. In: Dickson R, Harms J, eds. Modern Management of Spinal Deformities: A Theoretical, Practical, and Evidence-Based Text. 1st ed. Thieme; 2018).

 iii. Retract laryngeal mechanism, thyroid, and esophagus medially
 iv. Place Finochietto retractor and perform a manubrial split
  v. Insert nasogastric tube to identify cervical esophagus
 vi. Enter prevertebral space, exposing lower cervical and upper thoracic (a Weitlaner retractor can be inserted to enhance exposure)

b. T3–T10 approach (typically followed for thoracotomy):
   i. Enter chest two interspaces above the vertebrae of interest
   ii. Resect rib below incision (can be used in autograft if necessary)
   iii. Notch adjacent inferior rib to increase exposure
   iv. Utilize Bookwalter retraction system to retract chest wall, lung, and diaphragm
   v. Maintain rib separation with two shallow bladder blades and maintain downward traction on lung and diaphragm using deep straight blades

c. Thoracoabdominal approach (T11–L2):
   i. Resect the tenth rib and divide the ipsilateral hemidiaphragm circumferentially
   ii. Utilize Bookwalter retraction system to retract peritoneal contents and liver
   iii. Mobilize psoas musculature to access the vertebrae of interest

7. Once the vertebrae of interest are exposed, it is best to localize and verify the correct vertebrae via X-ray or fluoroscopic imaging and confirming with at least two people in the room

8. Perform the corpectomy for decompression over the desired segments based on preoperative imaging of levels that are compressed due to tumor

9. Place chest tube if significant pleural tear occurs (can be removed in 2–3 days)

10. After appropriate hemostasis is obtained, muscle and skin incisions can then be closed in appropriate fashion, often with placement of postoperative Jackson-Pratt drains that can be removed after 2 to 3 days

## Pitfalls

- Reduction in range of motion and mobility of fused spinal segments, if fusion is performed
- Intraoperative CSF leak
- Blood clot (deep vein thrombosis, or more severe pulmonary embolism)
- Damage to spinal nerves and/or cord
- Postoperative weakness or numbness or continued pain
- Postoperative wound infection
- Continued symptoms postsurgically/unresolved symptoms with no improvement to quality of life
- Prolonged hospitalization due to invasiveness of surgery and other comorbidities/iatrogenic infection
- Progressive kyphosis (see ▶ Fig. 2.26)
- Residual spinal compression
- Problems with bowel/bladder control

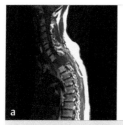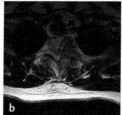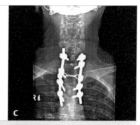

**Fig. 2.26** Radiology revealed a T5–T6 metastatic tumor in a middle-aged man (**a**). He received tumor resection treatment, radiotherapy, and chemotherapy, but the tumor expanded into the neural foramen, compressing the cord (**b**). It was resected via a posterolateral approach and the cord was stabilized by posterior segmental fixation (**c**). (Source: Operative technique and procedure. In: Dickman C, Fehlings M, Gokaslan Z, eds. Spinal Cord and Spinal Column Tumors. 1st ed. Thieme; 2006).

## Prognosis

- Hospitalization rates depend on the type of procedure performed, preoperative examination status, and patient's age/comorbidities
- Pain medications for postsurgical pain
- Physical therapy and occupational therapy will be needed postoperatively, immediately and as outpatient to regain strength
- Catheter placed in bladder and removed 1 to 2 days after surgery
- Brace placed after discharge for 8 weeks to immobilize to increase rate of healing

# Bibliography

Komanapalli C, Sukumar M. Thoracotomy for Exposure of the Spine. CTSNet. 2008. (https://www.ctsnet.org/article/thoracotomy-exposure-spine)

Lall RR, Smith ZA, Wong AP, Miller D, Fessler RG. Minimally invasive thoracic corpectomy: surgical strategies for malignancy, trauma, and complex spinal pathologies. Minim Invasive Surg 2012;2012:213791

Le HV, Wadhwa R, Mummaneni P, Theodore P. Anterior Transsternal Approach for Treatment of Upper Thoracic Vertebral Osteomyelitis: Case Report and Review of the Literature. Cureus 2015;7(9):e324

Paul RL, Michael RH, Dunn JE, Williams JP. Anterior transthoracic surgical decompression of acute spinal cord injuries. J Neurosurg 1975;43(3):299–307

Rangel-Castilla L, Russin JJ, Zaidi HA, et al. Contemporary management of spinal AVFs and AVMs: lessons learned from 110 cases. Neurosurg Focus 2014;37(3):E14

Schuchert MJ, McCormick KN, Abbas G, et al. Anterior thoracic surgical approaches in the treatment of spinal infections and neoplasms. Ann Thorac Surg 2014;97(5): 1750–1756, discussion 1756–1757

# 3 Lumbar

*Christ Ordookhanian and Paul E. Kaloostian*

## 3.1 Trauma

### 3.1.1 Lumbar Decompression with Foraminotomy/ Lumbar Diskectomy/Lumbar Fusion

#### Symptoms and Signs

- Paraplegia (incomplete or complete)
- Diminished control/dysfunction of bowel/bladder (including urinary retention) and external genitalia (men: problems with erection and ejaculation; women: problems with lubrication)
- Moderate/severe numbness in lower extremities and perianal area (saddle anesthesia)
- Paresthesia in lower body extremities
- Lower back/hip/pelvis/butt pain and loss of mobility due to the pain
- Muscle weakness in legs (paresis) or paralysis
- Radicular pain extending into legs
- Difficulty maintaining balance and walking
- Positive Babinski sign (in adults or children over 2 years old)
- Myelopathy
- Bruising of the lower back
- Hypotonia or flaccidity within 24 hours of injury
- Herniated disk(s)

#### Surgical Pathology

- Lumbar spine benign/malignant trauma

#### Diagnostic Modalities

- CT of lumbar spine without contrast
- CT myelography of lumbar spine
- MRI of lumbar spine without contrast
- X-ray of lumbar spine (to test for fractures; anterior–posterior and lateral views)
- CT or X-ray of hip/pelvis (not typically necessary)

# Differential Diagnosis

- Blunt trauma (complete and incomplete spinal cord injury [SCI])
- Penetrating trauma (complete and incomplete SCI)
- Wedge/Compression fracture
- Burst fracture
- Chance fracture
- Fracture-dislocation
- Compression fracture (most common of lumbar fractures)
- Ligamentous injury
- Musculoskeletal injury

# Treatment Options

- Acute pain control with medications and pain management
- Physical/Occupational/Rehabilitation therapy and rehabilitation
- If symptomatic with cord/nerve root compression:
  - Surgical decompression with or without fusion over implicated segments if deemed suitable candidate for surgery
    - If poor surgical candidate with poor life expectancy, medical management recommended
    - Surgery may be done anteriorly or posteriorly, or combined two-stage approach for added stabilization (typically only one stage needed posteriorly)
    - Foraminotomy (expanding space of neural foramen by removing soft tissues, small disk fragments, and bony spurs in the locus) (see ▶ Fig. 3.1)
    - Diskectomy (removal of section of herniated disk)
    - Endoscopic lumbar approach is minimally invasive and reduces complications (see ▶ Fig. 3.2)

# Indications for Surgical Intervention

- No improvement after nonoperative therapy (physical therapy, pain management)
- Residual spinal compression
- Unstable patterns of fracture
- Sufficient disruption of supporting ligaments
- Lumbar compression with posterior wall involvement and/or significant kyphosis
- Significant canal narrowing and/or significant kyphosis
- Neurologic dysfunction and/or instability resulting from lumbar trauma
  - Paresis or paralysis

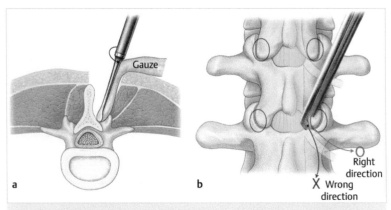

**Fig. 3.1 (a, b)** Illustration demonstrating midline open foraminotomy technique for addressing lumbar radiculopathy. (Source: Treatment option for LFSS. In: Kim D, Choi G, Lee S, et al, eds. Endoscopic Spine Surgery. 2nd ed. Thieme; 2018).

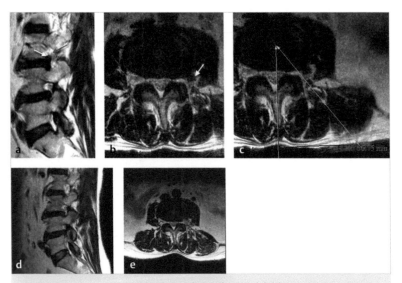

**Fig. 3.2 (a–e)** Preoperative MRI scan reveals extraforaminal disk herniation. Postoperative MRI scan demonstrates removal of herniated disk fragment in lumbar after employing an extraforaminal percutaneous endoscopic diskectomy approach. (Source: Percutaneous endoscopic lumbar diskectomy. In: Nader R, Berta S, Gragnanielllo C, et al, eds. Neurosurgery Tricks of the Trade: Spine and Peripheral Nerves. 1st ed. Thieme; 2014).

– Numbness in lower extremities and perianal area
– Bowel/Bladder dysfunction
- Clinical or radiographic instability

## Surgical Procedure for Posterior Lumbar Spine (Endoscopic Approach)

1. Informed consent signed, preoperative labs normal, no Aspirin/Plavix/Coumadin/NSAIDs/Advil/Celebrex/Ibuprofen/Motrin/Naprosyn/Aleve/other anticoagulants and anti-inflammatory drugs for at least 2 weeks
2. Appropriate intubation and sedation and lines (if necessary) as per the anesthetist (endotracheal delivery preferred)
3. Patient placed prone in neutral alignment on radiolucent table, enabling use of C-arm fluoroscope
4. Neuromonitoring not needed
5. Time out is performed with agreement from everyone in the room for correct patient and correct surgery with consent signed
6. Perform midline lumbar incision and dissect to lamina
7. Dissect lamina using lamina dissector through the working portal, under fluoroscopic guidance
8. Once the vertebrae of interest are exposed, it is best to localize and verify them via X-ray or fluoroscopic imaging and confirming with at least two people in the room
9. Perform foraminotomy:
   a. Dissect additional lamina and hypertrophied part of facet using endoscopic burr to expose the ligamentum flavum, controlling bleeding using radiofrequency coagulators
   b. Remove ligamentum flavum, thickened foraminal ligament, and bone spurs using micro punches and forceps, successfully exposing the exiting nerve root
   c. Coagulate the redundant disk and soft tissues compressing the nerve root using bipolar radiofrequency to relieve pressure from foraminal stenosis
10. Perform Diskectomy (if indicated in procedure):
    a. Retract the visible interfering nerve roots
    b. Incise through the indicated disk to expose large herniated disk fragment(s)
    c. Use a nerve hook to free them for removal
    d. Break adhesions between the herniated disk fragment(s) and surrounding structures to facilitate removal
    e. Using a grasper through the endoscopic apparatus, pull out the herniated disk fragment(s)

11. Remove lingering fragments as required
12. Ablate tissue debris using a side-firing laser
13. Remove remaining bone and ligament tissues using endoscopic punches
14. Mobilize exiting nerve root and dural sac under endoscopic visualization
15. Remove the endoscopic apparatus
16. Perform spinal fusion with instrumentation:
    a. Place open or percutaneous pedicle screws over segments involved with bone grafting to fuse these segments
    b. Insert small drainage catheter to reduce likelihood of postoperative epidural hematoma (can be removed after 2–3 days)
17. After appropriate hemostasis is obtained, muscle and skin incisions can then be closed in appropriate fashion

## Pitfalls

- Reduction in range of motion and mobility of fused spinal segments
- Intraoperative cerebrospinal fluid (CSF) leak
- Blood clot (deep vein thrombosis, or more severe pulmonary embolism)
- Damage to spinal nerves and/or cord (especially thecal sac injury and dural tear)
- Postoperative weakness or numbness or continued pain
- Postoperative wound infection
- Continued symptoms postsurgically/unresolved symptoms with no improvement to quality of life
- Loss of sensation
- Progressive kyphosis
- Residual spinal compression
- Problems with bowel/bladder control
- Epidural hematoma

## Prognosis

- Typically, no hospitalization (outpatient procedure), but hospitalization rates depend on the type of procedure performed, preoperative examination status, and patient's age/comorbidities
- Pain medications for postsurgical pain
- Physical therapy and occupational therapy will be needed postoperatively, immediately and as outpatient to regain strength
- Brace placed after discharge to immobilize to increase rate of healing

# 3.2 Elective

## 3.2.1 Lumbar Laminectomy/Decompression/Lumbar Diskectomy/Lumbar Synovial Cyst Resection/Lumbar Fusion Posterior

### Symptoms and Signs

- Degenerate spondylolisthesis
- Radiculopathy
- Neurogenic claudication
- Moderate numbness in lower extremities and perianal area (saddle anesthesia)
- Paresthesia in lower body extremities
- Lower back/hip/pelvis/butt pain and discomfort derived from consistent nerve irritation and loss of mobility due to the pain
- Muscle weakness in legs (paresis)
- Leg pain (sciatica)
- Difficulty maintaining balance and walking
- Muscle weakness and reduction of mobility from pain (as opposed to from nerve impairment, which typically requires emergent treatment, particularly if it relates to bladder function)
- Spinal instability

### Surgical Pathology

- Lumbar spine benign/malignant trauma
- Lumbar spine benign/malignant tumor
- Lumbar vascular benign/malignant lesion

### Diagnostic Modalities

- Clinical examination
- CT of lumbar spine with and without contrast
- CT myelography of lumbar spine
- MRI of lumbar spine with and without contrast
- CT or X-ray of hip/pelvis
- Angiography
- PET scan (search for tumor foci)
- Biopsy to examine tissue sample to determine whether tumor is benign or malignant, and what cancer type resulted in the tumor if malignancy is determined

# Differential Diagnosis

- Lumbar disk herniation
- Spinal stenosis (narrowing of the spine)
- Bulging lumbar disk
- Presence of synovial cyst or bone spurs (see ▸ Fig. 3.3)
- Tumor:
  - Metastatic (malignant, requiring emergent treatment)
  - Primary (benign or malignant)

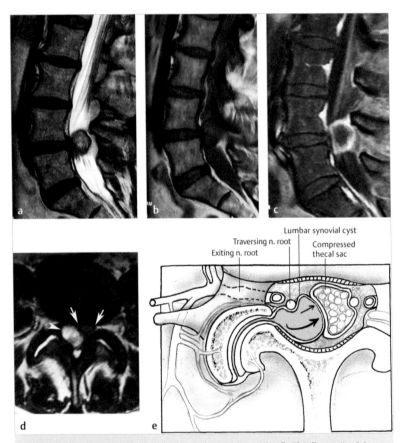

**Fig. 3.3** MRI scan revealed a lumbar synovial cyst at L4–L5 (**a–d**). The illustration (**e**) represents the MRI findings. (Source: Degenerative conditions. In: Khanna A, ed. MRI Essentials for the Spine Specialist. 1st ed. Thieme; 2014).

- Vascular lesion (typically requiring supplemental embolization):
  - Fibromuscular dysplasia (FMD)
  - Spinal arteriovenous malformation (AVM)
  - Spinal dural arteriovenous fistula (AVF)
- Vertebral trauma:
  - Blunt trauma (incomplete SCI)
  - Penetrating trauma (incomplete SCI)
  - Wedge/Compression fracture
  - Burst fracture
  - Chance fracture
  - Fracture-dislocation
  - Compression fracture
  - Ligamentous injury
  - Musculoskeletal injury

## Treatment Options

- Acute pain control with medications and pain management
- Physical/Occupational/Recreational therapy and rehabilitation
- If asymptomatic or mildly symptomatic with lumbar cord/nerve root compression and failed conservative routes:
  - Surgical decompression and fusion over implicated segments if deemed suitable candidate for surgery
    - If poor surgical candidate with poor life expectancy, medical management recommended
    - Surgery may be done anteriorly, posteriorly, or combined two-stage approach for added stabilization
    - May include a combination of the following techniques: Laminectomy (entire lamina, thickened ligaments, and part of enlarged facet joints removed to relieve pressure), Diskectomy (removal of section of herniated disk), synovial cyst removal
    - Endoscopic lumbar approach is minimally invasive and reduces complications

## Indications for Surgical Intervention

- Lumbar spinal stenosis (LSS)
- No sufficient improvement of pain and other symptoms after nonoperative measures (physical therapy, medications/injections, pain management)
- Disruption of supporting ligaments
- Lumbar compression

- Spinal condition isolated to specific locus of the body
- Significant reduction in everyday activities due to symptoms
- Expected postsurgical favorable outcome

## Surgical Procedure for Posterior Lumbar Spine (Endoscopic Approach)

1. Informed consent signed, preoperative labs normal, no Aspirin/Plavix/ Coumadin/NSAIDs/Advil/Celebrex/Ibuprofen/Motrin/Naprosyn/Aleve/ other anticoagulants and anti-inflammatory drugs for at least 2 weeks
2. Appropriate intubation and sedation and lines (if necessary) as per the anesthetist (endotracheal delivery preferred)
3. Patient placed prone in neutral alignment on radiolucent table, enabling use of C-arm fluoroscope
4. Neuromonitoring not needed
5. Time out is performed with agreement from everyone in the room for correct patient and correct surgery with consent signed
6. Perform midline incision over the appropriate level of interest based on X-ray and dissect to the spine
7. Confirm location on X-ray
8. Dissect lamina using lamina dissector through the working portal, under fluoroscopic guidance
9. Perform Laminotomy (see ▶ Fig. 3.4):
   a. Make small openings of the lamina, above and below the spinal nerve, using a drill
10. Perform Diskectomy:
    a. Retract the visible interfering nerve roots
    b. Incise through the indicated disk to expose large herniated disk fragment(s), under microscopic guidance
    c. Use a nerve hook to free them for removal
    d. Break adhesions between the herniated disk fragment(s) and surrounding structures to facilitate removal
    e. Using a grasper through the endoscopic apparatus, pull out the herniated disk fragment(s)
11. Perform synovial cyst resection:
    a. Resect the remaining visible interfering bone and ligamentum flavum, exposing the synovial cyst
    b. Sharply and bluntly dissect the synovial cyst, separating it from the dura
    c. Resect the synovial cyst
    d. Decompress the traversing nerve root medially and laterally

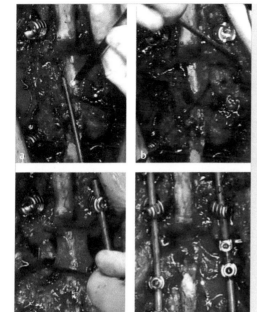

**Fig. 3.4** Intraoperative images of lumbar pedicle subtraction osteotomy. Laminectomy and facet resection are initially performed (**a**) and the osteotomy is closed with instrumentation (**d**). (Source: Surgical techniques. In: Ames C, Riew K, Abumi K, eds. Cervical Spine Deformity Surgery. 1st ed. Thieme; 2019).

12. Perform "clean-up" as necessary:
    a. Remove lingering fragments as required
    b. Ablate tissue debris using a side-firing laser
    c. Remove remaining bone and ligament tissues using endoscopic punches
13. Once the exiting nerve root and dural sac are mobilized, under endoscopic visualization, remove the endoscopic apparatus
14. Perform spinal fusion with instrumentation if instability or listhesis is present:
    a. Perform lumbar fusion if multiple vertebrae are involved, recurrent herniations occur, or spinal instability is significant
    b. Place percutaneous or open pedicle screws over segments involved with bone grafting, to fuse these segments
    c. Insert small drainage catheter to reduce likelihood of postoperative epidural hematoma (can be removed after 2–3 days)
15. After appropriate hemostasis is obtained, muscle and skin incisions can then be closed in appropriate fashion

## Pitfalls

- Reduction in range of motion and mobility of fused spinal segments
- Intraoperative CSF leak
- Blood clot (deep vein thrombosis, or more severe pulmonary embolism)
- Damage to spinal nerves and/or cord (especially thecal sac injury and dural tear)
- Postoperative weakness or numbness or continued pain
- Postoperative wound infection
- Prolonged hospitalization due to invasiveness of surgery and other comorbidities/iatrogenic infection
- Continued symptoms postsurgically/unresolved symptoms with no improvement to quality of life
- Loss of sensation
- Progressive kyphosis
- Residual spinal compression
- Problems with bowel/bladder control
- Recurrent disk herniation
- Epidural hematoma

## Prognosis

- Typically, no hospitalization (outpatient procedure), but hospitalization rates depend on the type of procedure performed, preoperative examination status, and patient's age/comorbidities; hospitalized patients are typically discharged after 1 to 2 days
- Pain medications for postsurgical pain
- Catheter placed in bladder and removed 1 to 2 days after surgery
- Physical therapy and occupational therapy will be needed postoperatively, immediately and as outpatient to regain strength
- Brace placed after discharge to immobilize to increase rate of healing

## 3.2.2 Anterior Lumbar Fusion

### Symptoms and Signs

- Moderate lower back/hip/pelvis/butt pain and reduction of mobility due to the pain
- Muscle weakness in legs (paresis)
- Difficulty maintaining balance and walking
- Spinal instability

- Muscle weakness and reduction of mobility from pain (as opposed to from nerve impairment, which typically requires emergent treatment, particularly if it relates to bladder function)

## Surgical Pathology

- Lumbar spine benign/malignant trauma
- Lumbar spine benign/malignant degenerative condition
- Lumbar spine benign/malignant postsurgical complication

## Diagnostic Modalities

- CT of lumbar spine without contrast
- MRI of lumbar spine without contrast
- X-ray of lumbar spine (to test for fractures; anterior–posterior and lateral views)
- CT or X-ray of hip/pelvis (not typically necessary)

## Differential Diagnosis

- Spondylolisthesis
- Degenerative disk disease
- Adjacent segment degeneration (ASD)
- Recurrent disk herniation
- Cage migration
- Pseudarthrosis

## Treatment Options

- Acute pain control with medications and pain management
- Physical/Occupational/Recreational therapy and rehabilitation
- If asymptomatic or mildly symptomatic with lumbar cord compression:
  - Surgical decompression and fusion over implicated segments if deemed suitable candidate for surgery
    - If poor surgical candidate with poor life expectancy, medical management recommended
    - Surgery may be done anteriorly, posteriorly, or combined two-stage approach for added stabilization
- If asymptomatic or mildly symptomatic without lumbar cord compression:
  - Surgical fusion over implicated segments if deemed suitable candidate for surgery
    - Posterior, anterior, and anterolateral approaches

## Indications for Surgical Intervention

- No sufficient improvement of pain and other symptoms after nonoperative measures (physical therapy, medications/injections, pain management)
- Spinal condition isolated to specific locus of the body
- Significant reduction in everyday and recreational activities due to symptoms
- Expected postsurgical favorable outcome

## Surgical Procedure for Anterior Lumbar Spine (Anterior Lumbar Interbody Fusion; ALIF)

1. Informed consent signed, preoperative labs normal, no Aspirin/Plavix/ Coumadin/NSAIDs/Advil/Celebrex/Ibuprofen/Motrin/Naprosyn/Aleve/ other anticoagulants and anti-inflammatory drugs for at least 2 weeks
2. Preoperative antibiotics delivered via IV injection
3. Appropriate intubation and sedation and lines (if necessary) as per the anesthetist (endotracheal tube and ventilator-assisted breathing)
4. Patient placed in supine position on radiolucent table, enabling use of C-arm fluoroscope
5. Place sterile drapes after properly cleansing the abdominal region
6. Neuromonitoring not needed
7. Time out is performed with agreement from everyone in the room for correct patient and correct surgery with consent signed
8. Make 3 to 8 cm transverse or oblique incision to the left of the belly button
9. Spread abdominal muscles apart without cutting them
10. Retract the peritoneal sac (including the intestines) and large blood vessels to the side
11. Visualize the anterior aspect of the intervertebral disks using retractors
12. Once the bone of interest is exposed, it is recommended to localize and verify it via fluoroscopic imaging and confirming with at least two people in the room
13. Remove the intervertebral disk using Pituitary rongeurs, Kerrison rongeurs, and curettes
14. Restore normal height of disk using distractor instruments and determine the size required for cage using fluoroscopy
15. Implant metal, plastic, or bone cage (with bone graft material) into the intervertebral disk space, under fluoroscopic guidance
16. Confirm that the location is correct using fluoroscopy

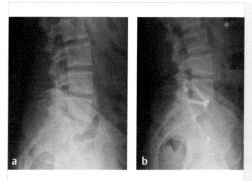

**Fig. 3.5** A middle-aged woman with discogenic lower back pain and a positive discogram at L5–S1 (**a**) received anterior lumbar interbody fusion (ALIF) and instrumentation for pain relief (**b**). (Source: Anterior lumbar interbody fusion (ALIF). In: Vaccaro A, Albert T, eds. Spine Surgery: Tricks of the Trade. 3rd ed. Thieme; 2016).

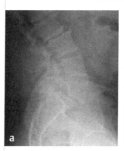
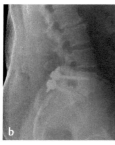

**Fig. 3.6** A middle-aged man with spondylolisthesis and back pain (**a**) received anterior lumbar interbody fusion (ALIF) and instrumentation at L5–S1 (**b**). (Source: Anterior lumbar interbody fusion (ALIF). In: Vaccaro A, Albert T, eds. Spine Surgery: Tricks of the Trade. 3rd ed. Thieme; 2016).

17. Add stability by adding instrumentation (a plate or pedicle screws to hold the cage in place) (see ▶ Fig. 3.5 and ▶ Fig. 3.6)
18. After appropriate hemostasis is obtained, muscle and skin incisions can then be closed in appropriate fashion

## Pitfalls

- Reduction in range of motion and mobility of fused spinal segments
- Intraoperative CSF leak
- Urethral injury
- Bowel perforation
- Incision hernia
- Ileus
- Retrograde ejaculation in men
- Vascular injury
- Damage to spinal nerves and/or cord

- Postoperative weakness or numbness or continued pain
- Postoperative wound infection
- Continued symptoms postsurgically/unresolved symptoms with no improvement to quality of life
- Loss of sensation

## Prognosis

- Hospitalization rates depend on the type of procedure performed, preoperative examination status, and patient's age/comorbidities
- Pain medications for postsurgical pain
- Physical therapy and occupational therapy will be needed postoperatively, immediately and as outpatient to regain strength
- Back brace placed after discharge to immobilize to increase rate of healing

# 3.2.3 Anterolateral Lumbar Fusion

## Symptoms and Signs

- Moderate lower back/hip/pelvis/butt pain and reduction of mobility due to the pain
- Muscle weakness in legs (paresis)
- Difficulty maintaining balance and walking
- Spinal instability
- Muscle weakness and reduction of mobility from pain (as opposed to from nerve impairment, which typically requires emergent treatment, particularly if it relates to bladder function)

## Surgical Pathology

- Lumbar spine benign/malignant trauma
- Lumbar spine benign/malignant degenerative condition
- Lumbar spine benign/malignant postsurgical complication

## Diagnostic Modalities

- CT of lumbar spine without contrast
- MRI of lumbar spine without contrast
- X-ray of lumbar spine (to test for fractures; anterior–posterior and lateral views)
- CT or X-ray of hip/pelvis (not typically necessary)

## Differential Diagnosis

- Spondylolisthesis
- Degenerative disk disease ASD
- Recurrent disk herniation
- Cage migration
- Pseudarthrosis

## Treatment Options

- Acute pain control with medications and pain management
- Physical/Occupational/Rehabilitation therapy and rehabilitation
- If asymptomatic or mildly symptomatic with lumbar cord compression:
  - Surgical decompression and fusion over implicated segments if deemed suitable candidate for surgery
    - If poor surgical candidate with poor life expectancy, medical management recommended
    - Surgery may be done anteriorly, anterolaterally, posteriorly, or combined two-stage approach for added stabilization
- If symptomatic and conservative routes failed with lumbar cord/nerve root compression:
  - Surgical fusion over implicated segments if deemed suitable candidate for surgery
    - Posterior, anterior, and anterolateral approaches

## Indications for Surgical Intervention

- No sufficient improvement of pain and other symptoms after nonoperative measures (physical therapy, medications/injections, pain management)
- Spinal condition isolated to specific locus of the body
- Significant reduction in everyday and recreational activities due to symptoms
- Expected postsurgical favorable outcome

## Surgical Procedure for Anterior Lumbar Spine (Anterolateral Lumbar Interbody Fusion; ALIF)

1. Informed consent signed, preoperative labs normal, no Aspirin/Plavix/Coumadin/NSAIDs/Advil/Celebrex/Ibuprofen/Motrin/Naprosyn/Aleve/other anticoagulants and anti-inflammatory drugs for at least 2 weeks

2. Preoperative antibiotics delivered via IV injection
3. Appropriate intubation and sedation and lines (if necessary) as per the anesthetist (endotracheal tube and ventilator-assisted breathing)
4. Patient placed in supine position on radiolucent table, enabling use of C-arm fluoroscope
5. Place sterile drapes after properly cleansing the lateral abdominal region
6. Neuromonitoring not needed
7. Time out is performed with agreement from everyone in the room for correct patient and correct surgery with consent signed
8. Make 4 to 6 cm transverse or oblique incision on the lateral abdomen wall, parallel to the projection of the disk level of interest (see ▶ Fig. 3.7)
9. Bluntly dissect the external and internal obliques and the transverse abdominal muscles
10. Mobilize the peritoneal content (including the intestines) inwardly
11. Bluntly separate the lateral edges of the iliac artery and vein from the spine using gentle, peanut sponge, and fingertip dissection
12. After medially retracting the large blood vessels and peritoneal contents, place hand-held abdominal retractor on anterolateral part of spine
13. Expose intervertebral disk of interest:
    a. If the vertebrae of interest are at or above L4–L5:
        i. Mobilize the psoas muscle and lumbar plexus

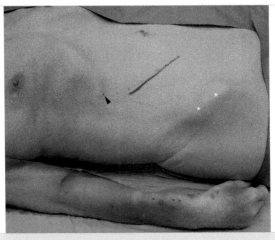

**Fig. 3.7** Image demonstrating incision to reveal lumbar plexus via an anterolateral extraperitoneal approach. Begin incision 4–5 cm below the *black arrowhead*. *White asterisks* mark the anterior superior iliac crest. (Source: Positioning and surgical exposure. In: Maniker A, ed. Operative Exposures in Peripheral Nerve Surgery. 1st ed. Thieme; 2004).

     ii. Place another hand-held abdominal retractor on the lateral side of the spine, retracting the psoas muscle and sympathetic nerves posteriorly, exposing the intervertebral disk between the aorta and psoas muscle

  b. If the vertebrae of interest are at L5–S1:

     i. Expose the intervertebral disk via two paths:

        ○ Below the aortic bifurcation

        ○ Over the aortic bifurcation's shoulder (between psoas muscle and left iliac artery)

14. Once the bone of interest is exposed, it is recommended to localize and verify it via fluoroscopic imaging and confirming with at least two people in the room

15. Perform diskectomy

16. Confirm complete decompression using a nerve hook

17. Prepare endplate using curettes

18. Remove the intervertebral disk using parallel distractor (Pituitary rongeurs, Kerrison rongeurs, or curettes)

19. Determine the size required for cage using fluoroscopy

20. Implant metal, plastic, or bone cage (with bone graft material) obliquely into the intervertebral disk space, under fluoroscopic guidance

21. Confirm that the location is correct using fluoroscopy

22. Add stability by adding instrumentation (a plate or pedicle screws to hold the cage in place, typically posterior instrumentation, and fusion is not necessary)

23. After appropriate hemostasis is obtained, muscle and skin incisions can then be closed in appropriate fashion

## Pitfalls

- Reduction in range of motion and mobility of fused spinal segments
- Intraoperative CSF leak
- Damage to spinal nerves and/or cord
- Postoperative weakness or numbness or continued pain
- Postoperative wound infection
- Continued symptoms postsurgically/unresolved symptoms with no improvement to quality of life
- Loss of sensation

## Prognosis

- Hospitalization rates depend on the type of procedure performed, preoperative examination status, and patient's age/comorbidities

- Pain medications for postsurgical pain
- Physical therapy and occupational therapy will be needed postoperatively, immediately and as outpatient to regain strength
- Back brace placed after discharge to immobilize to increase rate of healing

# 3.3 Tumor/Vascular

## 3.3.1 Lumbar Posterior Techniques for Tumor Resection (Vertebral Tumor)

### Symptoms and Signs

- Radicular pain extending into legs
- Diminished control/dysfunction of bowel/bladder (including urinary retention) and external genitalia (men: problems with erection and ejaculation; women: problems with lubrication)
- Moderate/Severe numbness in lower extremities and perianal area (saddle anesthesia)
- Paresthesia in lower body extremities
- Lower back/hip/pelvis/butt pain and loss of mobility due to the pain
- Muscle weakness in legs (paresis) or paralysis
- Leg pain (sciatica)
- Difficulty maintaining balance and walking
- Spinal instability
- Lower abdominal pain

### Surgical Pathology

- Lumbar spine benign/malignant tumor

### Diagnostic Modalities

- CT of lumbar spine with and without contrast to assess whether there is bony involvement of tumor
- MRI of lumbar spine with and without contrast to assess if there is spinal cord, epidural space, or nerve root involvement of tumor
- PET scan of body to look for other foci of tumor
- CT of chest/abdomen/pelvis to rule out metastatic disease and appendicitis
- Biopsy to examine tissue sample to determine whether tumor is benign or malignant, and what cancer type resulted in the tumor if malignancy is determined

## Differential Diagnosis

- Metastatic tumor
  - Breast, prostate, lung, renal cell
- Primary tumor
  - Intramedullary (typically reside in cervical or thoracic)
    - Astrocytoma
    - Ependymoma
    - Hemangioblastoma
    - Lipoma
  - Intradural extramedullary (see ▶ Fig. 3.8)

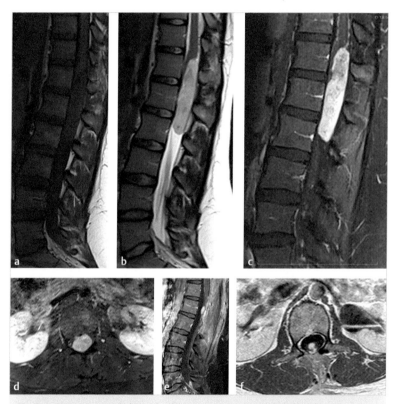

**Fig. 3.8** MRI scans revealed intradural tumor at T12–L2 (**a–d**). A subtotal piecemeal resection was performed, leaving residual tumor (**e, f**) which received radiation therapy. (Source: Extramedullary tumors of the spinal cord. In: Fessler R, Sekhar L, eds. Atlas of Neurosurgical Techniques: Spine and Peripheral Nerves. 2nd ed. Thieme; 2016).

- ○ Meningioma
- ○ Schwannoma
- ○ Neurofibroma
- ○ Ependymoma
- – Extradural (may reside within intervertebral foramen)

## Treatment Options

- Acute pain control with medications and pain management
- If asymptomatic or mildly symptomatic with lower body pain/radiculopathy with small focus of tumor:
  - – Radiation treatment (radiation oncology consultation)
    - ○ Some metastatic tumors are radioresistant
  - – Chemotherapy (medical oncology consultation)
    - ○ Some metastatic tumors are radioresistant
  - – Kyphoplasty (to treat pain)
  - – Surgical instrumentation and fusion (if there is concern for deformity, instability, or cord compression)
- If symptomatic with cord compression and myelopathy with large tumor burden:
  - – Urgent surgical decompression and fusion over multiple segments with tumor resection if deemed suitable candidate for surgery; may be followed by radiation treatment after resection if necessary as per the radiation oncologist:
    - ○ Oncologist will need to determine overall prognosis, Karnofsky performance score, and extent of visceral disease
    - ○ If poor surgical candidate with poor life expectancy, medical management recommended
    - ○ Surgery may be done anteriorly, posteriorly, or combined two-stage approach for added stabilization
  - – Preoperative embolization may be indicated for select vascular tumors to the spine such as renal cell cancer, thyroid cancer, breast cancer, etc. in order to decrease vascularity intraoperatively

## Indications for Surgical Intervention

- Spinal stenosis
- No improvement after nonoperative therapy (physical therapy, pain management, radiation treatment, and chemotherapy)
- Paraplegia
- Cord compression with or without myelopathy
- To obtain diagnosis if no other site for biopsy is available
- Risk of pathological fractures without stabilization

# Surgical Procedure for Posterior Lumbar Spine

1. Informed consent signed, preoperative labs normal, no Aspirin/Plavix/ Coumadin/NSAIDs/Advil/Celebrex/Ibuprofen/Motrin/Naprosyn/Aleve/ other anticoagulants and anti-inflammatory drugs for at least 2 weeks
2. Appropriate intubation and sedation and lines (if necessary) as per the anesthetist (endotracheal delivery preferred)
3. Patient placed prone in neutral alignment on radiolucent table, enabling use of C-arm fluoroscope
4. Neuromonitoring may be required to monitor nerves (if necessary and indicated)
5. Time out is performed with agreement from everyone in the room for correct patient and correct surgery with consent signed
6. Make two ipsilateral incisions in the paramedian area, 1 cm above and below the midsection of disk space in the lateral projection and on ipsilateral medial border of the pedicle in the anteroposterior projection
7. Insert serial dilators to create two portals, under fluoroscopic guidance
   a. If left approach, the left hole constitutes the endoscopic portal and the right hole constitutes the working portal
8. Dissect lamina using lamina dissector through the working portal, under fluoroscopic guidance
9. Once the vertebrae of interest are exposed, it is best to localize and verify them via X-ray or fluoroscopic imaging and confirming with at least two people in the room
10. Perform the laminectomy over the desired segments based on preoperative imaging of levels that are compressed due to tumor:
    a. Using Leksell rongeurs and hand-held high-speed drill, remove the bony spinous process and bilateral lamina as indicated for specific procedure
    b. Remove the thick ligamentum flavum with Kerrison rongeurs with careful dissection beneath the ligament to ensure no adhesions exist to dura mater below and thus avoiding CSF leak
    c. Perform appropriate foraminotomy with Kerrison rongeurs as needed for appropriate decompression of nerve roots
    d. Identify location of tumor and resect tumor as needed within the spinal canal:
       i. Use operative microscope and open the spinal cord dura midline with 11 blade and tack up the dural leaflets with suture
       ii. If tumor is intradural and extramedullary, the tumor can then be resected carefully with microdissection technique without cord injury (neuromonitoring needed in these cases)
       iii. If tumor is intradural and intramedullary, with microdissection technique the cord must be entered midline and the tumor must

be identified and resected starting centrally first, then around the edges (neuromonitoring needed in these cases)

11. After appropriate tumor resection, there may be need for additional stabilization to prevent kyphosis if the resection caused multiple segment decompression (see ▶ Fig. 3.9):
    a. Place percutaneous pedicle screws over segments involved with bone grafting to fuse these segments
    b. Insert small drainage catheter to reduce likelihood of postoperative epidural hematoma (can be removed after 2–3 days)

12. After appropriate hemostasis is obtained, muscle and skin incisions can then be closed in appropriate fashion, often with placement of postoperative drains that can be removed after 2 to 3 days

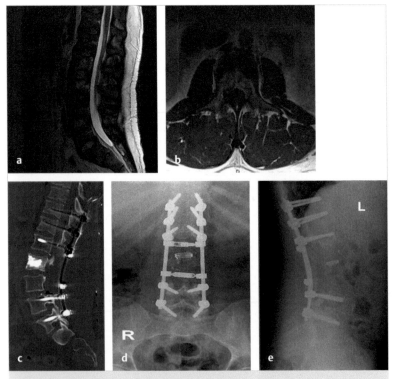

**Fig. 3.9 (a–e)** A middle-aged man with a chordoma at L2–L3 who already received proton beam radiation therapy underwent posterior L1–L4 laminectomy and T11–L5 fusion with instrumentation as well as L2–L3 spondylectomy and lumbar reconstruction from a left-side retroperitoneal approach. (Source: Surgery. In: Pamir M, Al-Mefty O, Borba L, eds. Chordomas: Technologies, Techniques, and Treatment Strategies. 1st ed. Thieme; 2017).

## Pitfalls

- Reduction in range of motion and mobility of fused spinal segments
- Intraoperative CSF leak
- Blood clot (deep vein thrombosis, or more severe pulmonary embolism)
- Damage to spinal nerves and/or cord (especially thecal sac injury and dural tear)
- Postoperative weakness or numbness or continued pain
- Postoperative wound infection
- Prolonged hospitalization due to invasiveness of surgery and other comorbidities/iatrogenic infection
- Continued symptoms postsurgically/unresolved symptoms with no improvement to quality of life
- Loss of sensation
- Progressive kyphosis
- Residual spinal compression
- Problems with bowel/bladder control
- Epidural hematoma

## Prognosis

- Typically, no hospitalization (outpatient procedure), but hospitalization rates depend on the type of procedure performed, preoperative examination status, and patient's age/comorbidities; hospitalized patients are typically discharged after 1 to 2 days
- Pain medications for postsurgical pain
- Catheter placed in bladder and removed 1 to 2 days after surgery
- Physical therapy and occupational therapy will be needed postoperatively, immediately and as outpatient to regain strength
- Brace placed after discharge to immobilize to increase rate of healing

## Pitfalls

- Reduction in range of motion and mobility of fused spinal segments
- Intraoperative CSF leak
- Urethral injury
- Bowel perforation
- Incision hernia
- Ileus
- Retrograde ejaculation in men
- Blood clot (deep vein thrombosis, or more severe pulmonary embolism)

- Damage to spinal nerves and/or cord
- Postoperative weakness or numbness or continued pain
- Postoperative wound infection
- Continued symptoms postsurgically/unresolved symptoms with no improvement to quality of life
- Loss of sensation

## Prognosis

- Hospitalization rates depend on the type of procedure performed, preoperative examination status, and patient's age/comorbidities
- Pain medications for postsurgical pain
- Physical therapy and occupational therapy will be needed postoperatively, immediately and as outpatient to regain strength
- Back brace placed after discharge to immobilize to increase rate of healing

### 3.3.2 Lumbar Anterior and Posterior Techniques for Vascular Lesion Treatment (Vertebral)

## Symptoms and Signs

- Dilated arteries and veins with dysplastic vessels
- Subarachnoid hemorrhage
- Myelopathy
- Seizure
- Ischemic injury to lumbar
- Increased sweating around lumbar vascular lesion
- Diminished control/dysfunction of bowel/bladder (including urinary retention) and external genitalia (men: problems with erection and ejaculation; women: problems with lubrication)
- Paresthesia in lower body extremities
- Difficulty maintaining balance and walking
- Lower back/hip/pelvis/butt pain and loss of mobility due to the pain
- Leg pain (sciatica)
- Moderate/Severe numbness in lower extremities and perianal area (saddle anesthesia)
- Muscle weakness in legs (paresis) or paralysis
- Spinal instability
- Lower abdominal pain
- Hemorrhaging

## Surgical Pathology

- Lumbar vascular benign/malignant lesions

## Diagnostic Modalities

- Angiography
  - Preoperative spinal angiography
  - Intraoperative indocyanine green (ICG) angiography
- CT of lumbar spine with and without contrast (can rule out acute hemorrhage)
- MRI of lumbar spine with and without contrast (see ▶ Fig. 3.10)

## Differential Diagnosis FMD

- Spinal AVM
  - Intradural-intramedullary (kemorrhaging common)
    - Glomus (Type II)
    - Juvenile (Type III)
  - Intradural-extramedullary
  - Conus medullaris
  - Metameric
  - Extradural
  - Cavernoma
  - Capillary telangiectasia
- Spinal dural AVF (Type I)
  - Intradural-extramedullary
    - Perimedullary AVF (Type IV)
  - Intradural-intramedullary
  - Extradural
- Vertebral sarcoidosis
- Dissection syndromes

## Treatment Options

- Conservative observation
- Radiation treatment
  - Conventional radiation (not very effective therapy)
  - Stereotactic radiosurgery and radiotherapy (nidus must not be greater than 3 cm in diameter)

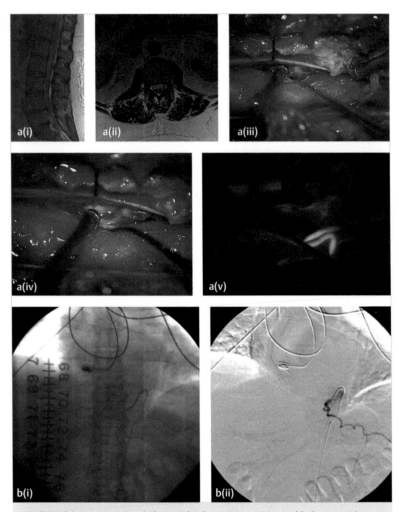

**Fig. 3.10** (a) MRI scans revealed an epidural mass at L1–L3 in an elderly man with lower back pain and paraplegia. The mass was resected with L1–L3 laminectomy. Intra-operatively, a thrombosed aneurysm of the artery of Adamkiewicz was discovered. (b) The aneurysm was resected to achieve cord decompression. (Source: Aneurysms of spinal arteries. In: Spetzler R, Kalani M, Nakaji P, eds. Neurovascular Surgery. 2nd ed. Thieme; 2015).

- Surgery
  - Microsurgical resection
  - Preferred option if bleeding or seizures result from lesion
- Endovascular embolization using the following embolic agents (initial procedure to facilitate surgery):
  - Coils: Close down vessel supplying AVM (cannot independently treat AVM nidus)
  - Onyx: Solidifies, forming a cast, in vessel supplying AVM (best penetration of AVM nidus)
  - N-butyl cyanoacrylate (tissue adhesive): Solidifies as a glue in vessel supplying AVM (greater risks and worse outcomes than with Onyx)
  - Polyvinyl alcohol: Used prior to craniotomy or surgical resection of AVM (cannot independently treat AVM pathology)
- Combination techniques
  - Embolization followed by stereotactic radiosurgery
- Venous angiomas should not be treated unless certainly contributing to intractable seizures and bleeding

## Indications for Endovascular Intervention

- Preoperative embolization (for surgical AVM resection)
- Presence of associated lesions (aneurysms/pseudoaneurysms on feeding pedicle or nidus, venous thrombosis, venous outflow restriction, venous pouches, dilatations)
- Small surgically inaccessible AVM treated by curative AVM embolization or radiosurgery
- Palliative treatment when symptomatic AVM not entirely treatable by the other approaches
- Paraplegia
- Cord compression with or without myelopathy

## Surgical Procedure for Posterior Lumbar Spine (Laminoplasty)

1. Administer 20 mg propranolol orally four times a day for 3 days to patient preoperation
2. Informed consent signed, preoperative labs normal, no Aspirin/Plavix/Coumadin/NSAIDs/Celebrex/Naprosyn/other anticoagulants and anti-inflammatory drugs for at least 2 weeks
3. Administer preoperative prophylactic IV antibiotics
4. Appropriate intubation and sedation and lines (if considered necessary by the anesthetist)

5. Patient placed prone on gel rolls, with head clamped via Mayfield Pins, pressure points padded, on radiolucent table, enabling use of C-arm fluoroscope
6. Neuromonitoring may be required to monitor nerves (if necessary and indicated)
7. Time out is performed with agreement from everyone in the room for correct patient and correct surgery with consent signed
8. Make an incision over the vertebrae where laminoplasty is to be performed:
    a. Prepare to utilize one level above and below the AVM nidus or AVF shunt
    b. Extension to ipsilateral pedicle performed if deemed necessary to enhance lateral exposure of the AVM nidus or AVF shunt
9. Inject local anesthetic into wound to lessen bleeding
10. Perform subperiosteal dissection of muscles bilaterally to expose the vertebra
11. Once the bone is exposed, it is best to localize and verify the correct vertebra via fluoroscopic imaging and confirming with at least two people in the room
12. Bovie electrocautery is used to progress dissection toward the spine and to attain hemostasis, with the help of bipolar forceps
13. Move musculature around vertebra laterally and downward to expose the dura
14. Utilize self-retaining retractors to keep everything in place
15. Open the dura, followed by the arachnoid
16. Clip the arachnoid to the dural edges using self-retaining retractors to reveal the vascular lesion source
17. Video-angiography (typically with ICG) is used to visualize the blood flow through the AVM
18. If the AVM nidus is intraparenchymal in its entirety, prepare to perform a myelotomy (midline dorsal, dorsal root entry zone, lateral, and anterior midline types). Otherwise, continue with the laminoplasty procedure (typically a pial resection).
19. Using the surgical suction and nonstick bipolar forceps, the pia arachnoid is revealed
20. Cut and coagulate the appropriate vessels
21. Separate AVM from the spinal cord using surgical scissors, bipolar, and suction
22. Several nerve rootlets will be tangled with the AVM (they may be tangled with dorsal nerve roots) and must be removed by necessity, others may be left unaltered
23. Cut the dentate ligament where it is attached to the AVM

24. The spinal canal is further exposed, revealing the feeders of the AVM
25. Use ICG video-angiography to confirm no further shunting of the arterial venous blood
26. Close the dura as well as the subcutaneous tissues after the laminoplasty is successfully performed
27. Close the skin with suture, skin-glue, steri-strips, or surgical staples
28. Postoperative injection of the relevant artery and vertebral locus demonstrate that the AVM has been treated

## Surgical Procedure for Anterior Lumbar Spine

1. Administer 20 mg propranolol orally four times a day for 3 days to patient preoperation
2. Informed consent signed, preoperative labs normal, no Aspirin/Plavix/Coumadin/NSAIDs/Celebrex/Naprosyn/other anticoagulants and anti-inflammatory drugs for at least 2 weeks
3. Administer preoperative prophylactic IV antibiotics
4. Appropriate intubation and sedation and lines (if necessary) as per the anesthetist (endotracheal tube and ventilator-assisted breathing)
5. Patient placed in supine position on radiolucent table, enabling use of C-arm fluoroscope
6. Place sterile drapes after properly cleansing the abdominal region
7. Neuromonitoring can be used
8. Time out is performed with agreement from everyone in the room for correct patient and correct surgery with consent signed
9. Make a 3 to 8 cm transverse or oblique incision to the left of the belly button
   a. Prepare to utilize one level above and below the AVM nidus or AVF shunt
   b. Extension to ipsilateral pedicle performed if deemed necessary to enhance lateral of the AVM nidus or AVF shunt
10. Spread abdominal muscles apart without cutting them
11. Retract the peritoneal sac (including the intestines) and large blood vessels to the side
12. Visualize the anterior aspect of the intervertebral disks using retractors
13. Once the bone of interest is exposed, it is recommended to localize and verify it via fluoroscopic imaging and confirming with at least two people in the room
14. Utilize self-retaining retractors to keep everything in place

15. If vertebral body contains tumor or other lesions, perform the anterior lumbar diskectomy or corpectomy at the appropriate level of lesion location with placement of cage and anterior plating
16. Obtain hemostasis and close wound in multiple layers

## Embolization Procedure (Onyx)

1. Shake Onyx vial on mixer for 20 minutes. Onyx-18 is common, Onyx-34 is suitable for very high flow AVMs, and Onyx-500 is incorporated in aneurysm embolization treatments
2. Wedge microcatheter tip into arterial branch supplying the AVM, preferably very close to the AVM nidus
3. Perform angiography through the microcatheter to confirm that the arterial branch exclusively supplies the AVM
4. Prime the DMSO-compatible microcatheter (marathon, echelon, rebar, ultra flow) with 0.3 to 0.8 mL DMSO so that Onyx does not solidify in the microcatheter
5. Slowly inject Onyx solution, allowing no more than 1 cm of reflux. If reflux occurs, continue after 1 to 2 minute waiting period
6. Halt injection when Onyx no longer flows into the nidus, but refluxes instead

## Pitfalls

- Stroke
- Intraoperative and postoperative bleeding
- Failure to remove entire vascular lesion source
- Future recurrence of vascular lesion
- Recompression of lumbar spinal cord
- Postlaminoplasty kyphosis
- Nerve root palsies
- Damage to spinal nerves and/or cord
- Postoperative weakness or numbness or continued pain
- Postoperative wound infection
- Prolonged hospitalization due to invasiveness of surgery and other comorbidities/iatrogenic infection
- Temporary postoperative paresthesia
- Iatrogenic vertebral artery injury during embolization process

## Prognosis

- Admit patient to intensive care unit (ICU)
- Keep leg on the side used during procedure straight for 2 hours (if angioseal closure) or 6 to 8 hours (if manual compression), keeping head of bed elevated by 15 degrees
- Check groins, DP's, vitals, and neuro checks q 15 min ×4, q 30 min ×4, then q hr
- Maintain mild hypotension 12 to 72 hours postoperative
- Monitor patient for perfusion pressure break through bleeding, seizures, and other possible complications
- Review/resume preprocedure medications (hold metformin 48 hours postprocedure; hold oral hypoglycemics until satisfactory oral intake)
- Schedule outpatient appointment 4 weeks postprocedure
- Angiography (not CTA or MRA) 1 and 5 years postprocedure (AVM), or MRI 3 months postprocedure, depending on the cause of lesion (spinal cavernous malformations)

## 3.3.3 Lumbar Anterior and Posterior Techniques for Tumor Resection (Spinal Canal Pathology)

### Symptoms and Signs

- Incidental with symptoms (depending on size and location)
- Diminished control/dysfunction of bowel/bladder (including urinary retention) and external genitalia (men: problems with erection and ejaculation; women: problems with lubrication)
- Moderate/Severe numbness in lower extremities and perianal area (saddle anesthesia)
- Paresthesia in lower body extremities
- Lower back/hip/pelvis/butt pain and loss of mobility due to the pain
- Muscle weakness in legs (paresis) or paralysis
- Leg pain (sciatica)
- Difficulty maintaining balance and walking
- Spinal instability
- Lower abdominal pain

### Surgical Pathology

- Lumbar spine benign/malignant tumor

## Diagnostic Modalities

- CT of lumbar spine with and without contrast to assess whether there is bony involvement of tumor
- MRI of lumbar spine with and without contrast to assess if there is spinal cord, epidural space, or nerve root involvement of tumor
- PET scan of body to look for other foci of tumor
- CT of chest/abdomen/pelvis to rule out metastatic disease and appendicitis
- X-ray (not as reliable for tumor diagnosis)
- Biopsy to examine tissue sample to determine whether tumor is benign or malignant, and what cancer type resulted in the tumor if malignancy is determined

## Differential Diagnosis

- Metastatic tumor
  - Breast, prostate, lung, renal cell
- Primary tumor
  - Intramedullary (typically reside in cervical or thoracic)
    - Astrocytoma
    - Ependymoma
    - Hemangioblastoma
    - Lipoma (see ▶ Fig. 3.11)
  - Intradural extramedullary (see ▶ Fig. 3.12)
    - Meningioma
    - Schwannoma
    - Neurofibroma
    - Ependymoma
  - Extradural (may reside within intervertebral foramen)

## Treatment Options

- Acute pain control with medications and pain management
- If asymptomatic or mildly symptomatic with lower body pain/radiculopathy with small focus of tumor:
  - Radiation treatment (radiation oncology consultation)
    - Some metastatic tumors are radioresistant
  - Chemotherapy (medical oncology consultation)
    - Some metastatic tumors are radioresistant
  - Kyphoplasty (to treat pain)
  - Surgical instrumentation and fusion (if there is concern for deformity, instability, or cord compression)

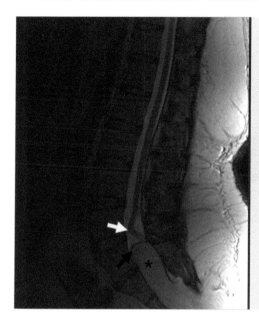

**Fig. 3.11** MRI scan reveals a lower lumbar lipoma extending into the spinal canal (*asterisk*). (Source: Case 120: a patient with urinary incontinence and a subcutaneous mass in the sacral region. In: Riascos R, Bonfante E, Calle S, eds. RadCases Plus Q&A: Neuro Imaging. 2nd ed. Thieme; 2018).

- If symptomatic with cord compression and myelopathy with large tumor burden:
  - Urgent surgical decompression and fusion over multiple segments with tumor resection if deemed suitable candidate for surgery; may be followed by radiation treatment after resection if considered necessary by the radiation oncologist:
    - Oncologist will need to determine overall prognosis, Karnofsky performance score, and extent of visceral disease
    - If poor surgical candidate with poor life expectancy, medical management recommended
    - Surgery may be done anteriorly, posteriorly, or combined two-stage approach for added stabilization if necessary
  - Preoperative embolization may be indicated for select vascular tumors to the spine such as renal cell cancer, thyroid cancer, breast cancer, etc. in order to decrease vascularity intraoperatively

## Indications for Surgical Intervention

- Spinal stenosis
- No improvement after nonoperative therapy (physical therapy, pain management)

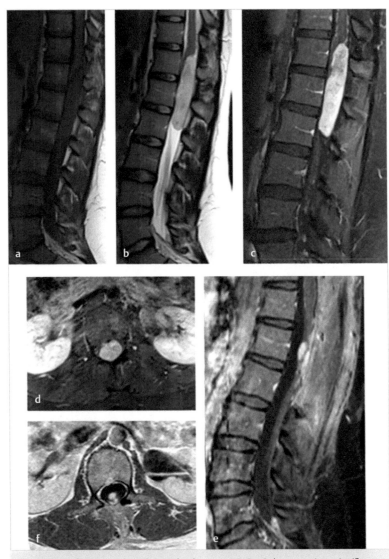

**Fig. 3.12 (a–f)** MRI scan reveals intradural tumor at T12–L2 that occupies a significant portion of the spinal canal. A subtotal piecemeal resection was performed along with radiation therapy to address residual tumor. (Source: Extramedullary tumors of the spinal cord. In: Fessler R, Sekhar L, eds. Atlas of Neurosurgical Techniques: Spine and Peripheral Nerves. 2nd ed. Thieme; 2016).

- Paraplegia
- Cord/Central canal compression with or without myelopathy
- To obtain diagnosis if no other site for biopsy is available
- Risk of pathological fractures without stabilization

## Surgical Procedure for Posterior Lumbar Spine

1. Informed consent signed, preoperative labs normal, no Aspirin/Plavix/Coumadin/NSAIDs/Advil/Celebrex/Ibuprofen/Motrin/Naprosyn/Aleve/other anticoagulants and anti-inflammatory drugs for at least 2 weeks
2. Appropriate intubation and sedation and lines (if necessary) as per the anesthetist (endotracheal delivery preferred)
3. Patient placed prone in neutral alignment on radiolucent table, enabling use of C-arm fluoroscope
4. Neuromonitoring may be required to monitor nerves (if necessary and indicated for intradural tumors only)
5. Time out is performed with agreement from everyone in the room for correct patient and correct surgery with consent signed
6. Make two ipsilateral incisions in the paramedian area, 1 cm above and below the midsection of disk space in the lateral projection and on ipsilateral medial border of the pedicle in the anteroposterior projection
7. Insert serial dilators to create two portals, under fluoroscopic guidance
   a. If left approach, the left hole constitutes the endoscopic portal and the right hole constitutes the working portal
8. Dissect lamina using lamina dissector through the working portal, under fluoroscopic guidance
9. Prepare endoscopic apparatus
   a. Send guide wire, under fluoroscopic guidance, to extraforaminal zone at the vertebrae of interest
   b. Muscles are preferably moved aside rather than cut, when possible
   c. Insert tapered dilator over guide wire
   d. Insert portal tube over tapered dilator
      i. The exiting nerve end, traveling through the intervertebral foramen, is protected by the tapered end of the portal tube
   e. Place endoscope through the portal tube, exposing the superior facet, to identify bone overgrowth
   f. Use endoscopic irrigation system to drain the irrigation fluid from the endoscopic portal to the working portal (a retractor or tube is not necessary for directing the flow of drainage)
10. Once the vertebrae of interest are exposed, it is recommended to localize and verify them via X-ray or fluoroscopic imaging and confirming with at least two people in the room

11. Perform the laminectomy over the desired segments based on preoperative imaging of levels that are compressed due to tumor:
    a. Using Leksell rongeurs and hand-held high-speed drill, remove the bony spinous process and bilateral lamina as indicated for specific procedure
    b. Remove the thick ligamentum flavum with Kerrison rongeurs with careful dissection beneath the ligament to ensure no adhesions exist to dura mater below and thus avoiding CSF leak
    c. Perform appropriate foraminotomy with Kerrison rongeurs as needed for appropriate decompression of nerve roots
    d. Identify location of tumor and resect tumor as needed within the spinal canal
        i. Use operative microscope and open the spinal cord dura midline with size 11 blade and tack up the dural leaflets with suture
        ii. If tumor is intradural and extramedullary, the tumor can then be resected carefully with microdissection technique without cord injury (neuromonitoring needed in these cases)
        iii. Once adhesions between the tumor and surrounding structures are sufficiently disrupted, a grasper can be used through the endoscopic apparatus to pull out tumor components
12. After appropriate tumor resection, there may be need for additional stabilization to prevent kyphosis if the resection caused multiple segment decompression: (see ▶ Fig. 3.9)
    a. Place percutaneous pedicle screws over segments involved with bone grafting to fuse these segments
    b. Insert small drainage catheter to reduce likelihood of postoperative epidural hematoma (can be removed after 2–3 days)
13. After appropriate hemostasis is obtained, muscle and skin incisions can then be closed in appropriate fashion, often with placement of postoperative drains that can be removed after 2 to 3 days

## Pitfalls

- Reduction in range of motion and mobility of fused spinal segments
- Intraoperative CSF leak
- Blood clot (deep vein thrombosis, or more severe pulmonary embolism)
- Damage to spinal nerves and/or cord (especially thecal sac injury and dural tear)
- Postoperative weakness or numbness or continued pain
- Postoperative wound infection
- Prolonged hospitalization due to invasiveness of surgery and other comorbidities/iatrogenic infection
- Continued symptoms postsurgically/unresolved symptoms with no improvement to quality of life

- Loss of sensation
- Progressive kyphosis
- Residual spinal compression
- Problems with bowel/bladder control
- Epidural hematoma

## Prognosis

- Typically, no hospitalization (outpatient procedure), but hospitalization rates depend on the type of procedure performed, preoperative examination status, and patient's age/comorbidities; hospitalized patients are typically discharged after 1 to 2 days
- Pain medications for postsurgical pain
- Physical therapy and occupational therapy will be needed postoperatively, immediately and as outpatient to regain strength
- Brace placed after discharge to immobilize to increase rate of healing

## Surgical Procedure for Anterior Lumbar Spine

1. Informed consent signed, preoperative labs normal, no Aspirin/Plavix/Coumadin/NSAIDs/Advil/Celebrex/Ibuprofen/Motrin/Naprosyn/Aleve/other anticoagulants and anti-inflammatory drugs for at least 2 weeks
2. Preoperative antibiotics delivered via IV injection
3. Appropriate intubation and sedation and lines (if necessary) as per the anesthetist (endotracheal tube and ventilator-assisted breathing)
4. Patient placed in supine position on radiolucent table, enabling use of C-arm fluoroscope
5. Place sterile drapes after properly cleansing the abdominal region
6. Neuromonitoring not needed
7. Time out is performed with agreement from everyone in the room for correct patient and correct surgery with consent signed
8. Make 3 to 8 cm transverse or oblique incision to the left of the belly button
9. Spread abdominal muscles apart without cutting them
10. Retract the peritoneal sac (including the intestines) and large blood vessels to the side
11. Visualize the anterior aspect of the intervertebral disks using retractors
12. Once the bone of interest is exposed, it is recommended to localize and verify it via fluoroscopic imaging and confirming with at least two people in the room
13. After appropriate tumor resection, there may be need for additional stabilization to prevent kyphosis if the resection caused multiple segment decompression. Therefore, perform instrumentation by placing anterior cage for reconstruction with anterior plating

14. After appropriate hemostasis is obtained, muscle and skin incisions can then be closed in appropriate fashion, often with placement of postoperative Jackson-Pratt drains that can be removed after 2 to 3 days

## Pitfalls

- Reduction in range of motion and mobility of fused spinal segments
- Intraoperative CSF leak
- Urethral injury
- Bowel perforation
- Incision hernia
- Ileus
- Retrograde ejaculation in men
- Blood clot (deep vein thrombosis, or more severe pulmonary embolism)
- Damage to spinal nerves and/or cord
- Postoperative weakness or numbness or continued pain
- Postoperative wound infection
- Continued symptoms postsurgically/unresolved symptoms with no improvement to quality of life
- Loss of sensation

## Prognosis

- Hospitalization rates depend on the type of procedure performed, preoperative examination status, and patient's age/comorbidities
- Pain medications for postsurgical pain
- Physical therapy and occupational therapy will be needed postoperatively, immediately and as outpatient to regain strength
- Back brace placed after discharge to immobilize to increase rate of healing

# Bibliography

Heo DH, Son SK, Eum JH, Park CK. Fully endoscopic lumbar interbody fusion using a percutaneous unilateral biportal endoscopic technique: technical note and preliminary clinical results. Neurosurg Focus 2017;43(2):E8

Kuang L, Chen Y, Li L, Lü G, Wang B. Applying the mini-open anterolateral lumbar interbody fusion with self-anchored stand-alone polyetheretherketone cage in lumbar revision surgery. BioMed Res Int 2016;2016:1758352

Rangel-Castilla L, Russin JJ, Zaidi HA, et al. Contemporary management of spinal AVFs and AVMs: lessons learned from 110 cases. Neurosurg Focus 2014;37(3):E14

Schizas C, Mouhsine E, Chevalley F, Theumann N, Duff J. [Surgical indications in spinal trauma] Rev Med Suisse 2005;1(46):2978–2981

Sherman AL, Kishner S. Lumbar Compression Fracture Treatment & Management. Medscape. 2018. (https://emedicine.medscape.com/article/309615-treatment)

# 4 Sacral

*Christ Ordookhanian and Paul E. Kaloostian*

## 4.1 Trauma

### 4.1.1 Sacral Fusion

#### Symptoms and Signs

- Diminished control/dysfunction of bladder/bowel, rectum, urinary system, and external genitalia (men: problems with erection and ejaculation; women: problems with lubrication)
- Moderate/Severe numbness in perianal area (saddle anesthesia)
- Loss of sensation along S2–S5 dermatomes
- Muscle weakness in perianal/perineal region, including difficulty in voluntarily contracting the anus
- Moderate/Severe pain in the sacral region (including peripelvic pain)
- Bruising of the pelvic and buttocks regions
- Pelvic ring injury
- Spondylolisthesis
- Cauda equina symptoms
- Deficits in lower extremities
- Refractory lower back pain

#### Surgical Pathology

- Sacral spine benign/malignant trauma

#### Diagnostic Modalities

- Physical/Neurologic examination and patient history
- CT of sacrum without contrast (coronal and sagittal reconstruction views)
- MRI of sacrum without contrast (when neural compromise may be indicated)
- X-ray of sacrum (best views: AP, lateral, inlet, and outlet)
- CT or X-ray of pelvis (not typically necessary)

#### Differential Diagnosis

- Zone 1 fracture (lateral to foramina)
  - Most common

- Zone 2 fracture (through foramina)
  – Very unstable with shear component
- Zone 3 fracture (medial to foramina into spinal canal)
  – Frequently results in neurologic deficit
- Transverse fracture
  – Frequently results in nerve dysfunction
- U-type fracture
  – Frequently results in neurologic deficit

## Treatment Options

- Acute pain control with medications and pain management
- Physical/Occupational/Rehabilitation therapy and rehabilitation
  – Progressive weight bearing with or without orthosis (if no neurologic deficit and little displacement)
- If symptomatic without neurologic injury:
  – Urgent surgical fixation of implicated segments if deemed suitable candidate for surgery
    ◦ If poor surgical candidate with poor life expectancy, medical management recommended
    ◦ Percutaneous screw fixation
    ◦ Posterior tension band plating
    ◦ Iliosacral and lumbopelvic fixation
- If symptomatic with cord compression:
  – Urgent surgical decompression and fusion of implicated segments if deemed suitable candidate for surgery
    ◦ If poor surgical candidate with poor life expectancy, medical management recommended
    ◦ Surgery may be done indirectly through axial traction or directly (posteriorly)
    ◦ May include a combination of the following techniques: Laminectomy (entire lamina, thickened ligaments, and part of enlarged facet joints removed to relieve pressure), Laminotomy (section of lamina and ligament removed), Foraminotomy (expanding space of neural foramen by removing soft tissues, small disk fragments, and bony spurs in the locus), Laminoplasty (expanding space within spinal canal by repositioning lamina), Diskectomy (removal of section of herniated disk), Corpectomy (removal of vertebral body and disks), Bony Spur Removal
    ◦ This may be accompanied by fusion for added stabilization (see ▶ Fig. 4.1)

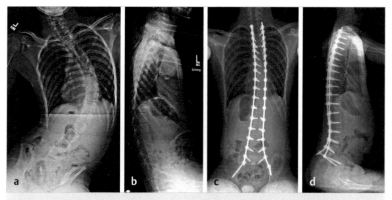

**Fig. 4.1** A teenage boy who suffered a complete spinal cord injury, accompanied by severe kyphosis (**a**, **b**), received a posterior spinal fusion with instrumentation at T2-Sacrum/Pelvis (**c**, **d**). (Source: Prevalence. In: Samdani A, Newton P, Sponseller P, et al, eds. Neuromuscular Spine Deformity: A Harms Study Group Treatment Guide. 1st ed. Thieme; 2018).

## Indications for Surgical Intervention

- No improvement after nonoperative therapy (physical therapy, pain management)
- Fracture displacement greater than 1 cm
- Fracture displacement after nonoperative therapy
- Soft tissue is compromised
- Unstable patterns of fracture
- Neurologic dysfunction and/or instability resulting from sacral trauma

## Surgical Procedure for Posterior Sacral Spine (Instrumentation without Fusion)

1. Informed consent signed, preoperative labs normal, no Aspirin/Plavix/ Coumadin/NSAIDs/Advil/Celebrex/Ibuprofen/Motrin/Naprosyn/Aleve/ other anticoagulants and anti-inflammatory drugs for at least 2 weeks
2. Appropriate intubation and sedation and lines (if necessary) as per the anesthetist
3. Patient placed prone on OSI spine table, with pillows placed under thighs
4. Neuromonitoring not needed
5. Apply bifemoral skeletal traction

    a. Femoral traction can be applied in two ways:
        i. Traction bow posterior to thighs (extends pelvis and reduces kyphotic deformity)
        ii. Traction bow anterior to thighs (longitudinal traction, reducing traumatic spondyloptosis)

6. Visualize the sacral fracture using fluoroscopy
    a. Traction is applied to reduce it

7. Prepare pedicle screws placement into L4 and L5 (bilateral percutaneous pedicle screws with 6–7 mm diameters; four in total):
    a. Make 2 to 3 cm bilateral incisions above the L4 and L5 levels of vertebrae, 1 to 2 cm lateral to the lateral L4 and L5 pedicle walls
    b. Insert introducer needles and subsequently place guide wires, under fluoroscopic guidance
    c. Hold the guide wires out of the way using hemostats

8. Place iliac screws (bilateral iliac screws with 8–9 mm diameters and 80–100 mm lengths; two in total):
    a. Make 2 cm bilateral incisions, at the level of and 0.1 to 1 cm medial to posterior superior iliac spine (PSIS)
    b. Perform sharp dissection to expose fascia on the iliac crest
    c. Split fascia longitudinally over iliac crest using electrocautery, halfway between medial and lateral border, and elevate it off the medial side
    d. Perform digital dissection to elevate the muscle off the medial side of iliac crest and expose the posterior sacral cortex (use retractors as necessary)
    e. Remove sufficient iliac bone, including medial part of dorsal cortex, using gouges, to place iliac screws and provide enough room for the rods
    f. Use curved tip of blunt curved probe, in conjunction with fluoroscopic imaging, to confirm the trajectory of screw placement
    g. Place the iliac screws through the established pathway, continuing until the screw heads make contact with the sacrum

9. Sufficient proximal and distal clearance across the iliac crest bone from the iliac screws must be made in preparation for rod placement, using a straight osteotome
    a. Bilateral rods (two in total) with 5.5 mm diameters are used
    b. Once accomplished, place pedicle screws over the previously established guidewires

10. Reduce the fracture:
    a. Reduce the fracture using direct manipulation of the iliac screws, by handling the left-in-place screws with insertion drivers
    b. Hold the fracture in place through the screws on one side of spine, while removing screwdrivers on other side of spine

c. Pass the rod and place set screws, tightening them
d. Remove the contralateral screwdrivers and pass the other rod, placing and tightening the remaining set screws
e. When the rod is placed into the L4 and L5 screws, the iliac screw heads pivot
f. Tighten the iliac screws

11. After appropriate hemostasis is obtained, muscle and skin incisions can then be closed in appropriate fashion
12. Instrumentation can be removed 4 to 6 months after surgery after the healing of the fracture is confirmed via CT

## Pitfalls

- Intraoperative cerebrospinal (CSF) leak
- Damage to spinal nerves and/or cord (especially thecal sac injury and dural tear)
- Postoperative weakness or numbness or continued pain
- Postoperative wound infection
- Continued symptoms postsurgically/unresolved symptoms with no improvement to quality of life
- Progressive kyphosis
- Problems with bowel/bladder control
- Venous thromboembolism (frequently from immobility)
- Iatrogenic nerve injury (frequently from fracture overcompression)
- Malreduction (frequently associated with vertically displaced fractures)

## Surgical Procedure for Anterior Sacral Spine (Anterior Lumbar Interbody Fusion with Transperitoneal Approach)

1. Informed consent signed, preoperative labs normal, no Aspirin/Plavix/ Coumadin/NSAIDs/Advil/Celebrex/Ibuprofen/Motrin/Naprosyn/Aleve/ other anticoagulants and anti-inflammatory drugs for at least 2 weeks
2. Preoperative antibiotics delivered via IV injection
3. Appropriate intubation and sedation and lines (if necessary) as per the anesthetist (endotracheal tube and ventilator-assisted breathing)
4. Patient placed in supine position on radiolucent table, enabling use of C-arm fluoroscope
5. Place sterile drapes after properly cleansing the abdominal region
6. Neuromonitoring not needed
7. Time out is performed with agreement from everyone in the room for correct patient and correct surgery with consent signed

8. Make midline abdominal skin incision over the L5–S1 level
9. Open the linea alba by performing another midline incision
10. Spread abdominal muscles apart without cutting them
11. Retract the peritoneal sac (including the intestines) and large blood vessels to the left side using retractors
12. Visualize the anterior aspect of the intervertebral disks using retractors
13. Once the bone of interest is exposed, it is recommended to localize and verify it via fluoroscopic imaging and confirming with at least two people in the room
14. Remove the intervertebral disk using Pituitary rongeurs, Kerrison rongeurs, and curettes (diskectomy)
15. Restore normal height of disk using distractor instruments and determine the size required for cage using fluoroscopy
16. Implant metal, plastic, or bone cage (with bone graft material) into the intervertebral disk space, under fluoroscopic guidance
17. Confirm that the location is correct using fluoroscopy
18. Add stability by adding instrumentation (a plate or screws/rods to hold the cage in place)
19. After appropriate hemostasis is obtained, muscle and skin incisions can then be closed in appropriate fashion

## Pitfalls

- Reduction in range of motion and mobility of fused spinal segments
- Intraoperative CSF leak
- Urethral injury
- Bowel perforation
- Incision hernia
- Ileus
- Retrograde ejaculation in men
- Vascular injury
- Damage to spinal nerves and/or cord
- Postoperative weakness or numbness or continued pain
- Postoperative wound infection

## Prognosis

- Hospitalization rates depend on the type of procedure performed, preoperative examination status, and patient's age/comorbidities
- Pain medications for postsurgical pain
- Physical therapy and occupational therapy will be needed postoperatively, immediately and as outpatient to regain strength
- Brace placed after discharge to immobilize to increase rate of healing

## 4.1.2 Tarlov Cyst Treatment

### Symptoms and Signs

- Diminished control/dysfunction of bladder/bowel, rectum, urinary system, and external genitalia (men: problems with erection and ejaculation; women: problems with lubrication)
- Moderate/Severe numbness in perianal area (saddle anesthesia)
- Loss of sensation along S2–S5 dermatomes
- Muscle weakness in perianal/perineal region, including difficulty in voluntarily contracting the anus
- Moderate/Severe pain in the sacral region (including peripelvic pain)
- Bruising of the pelvic and buttocks regions
- Pelvic ring injury
- Spondylolisthesis
- Cauda equina symptoms
- Deficits in lower extremities
- Refractory lower back pain
- Radicular pain in lower body
- Sciatica
- Impaired reflexes
- Coccydynia

### Surgical Pathology

- Sacral spine benign/malignant cyst
- Sacral spine benign/malignant trauma

### Diagnostic Modalities

- Physical/Neurologic examination and patient history
- CT myelography
- MRI of lumbosacral spine without contrast (when neural compromise may be indicated) (see ▶ Fig. 4.2)
- X-ray of sacrum (best views: AP, lateral, inlet, and outlet)
- CT or X-ray of pelvis (not typically necessary)
- Urological testing (urodynamics, cystoscopy, kidney ultrasound)

### Differential Diagnosis

- Fracture
  - Zone 1 fracture (lateral to foramina)
    - Most common

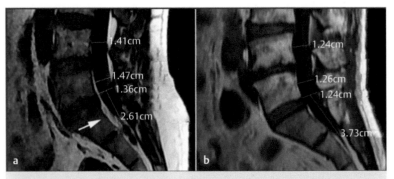

**Fig. 4.2** An MRI scan demonstrating a sacral Tarlov cyst (**a**) is compared with a control lumbosacral MRI (**b**). (Source: Xie C, Zheng X, Zhang N. Tarlov cyst is correlated with a short broad terminal of the thecal sac. J Neurol Surg A Cent Eur Neurosurg 2017;78(3):245–249).

- – Zone 2 fracture (through foramina)
  - ○ Very unstable with shear component
- – Zone 3 fracture (medial to foramina into spinal canal)
  - ○ Frequently results in neurologic deficit
- – Transverse fracture
  - ○ Frequently results in nerve dysfunction
- – U-type fracture
  - ○ Frequently results in neurologic deficit
- • Tarlov cyst (see ▶ Fig. 4.3)
- • Disk herniation(s)
- • Gynecological conditions
- • Meningeal diverticula
- • Meningoceles
- • Arachnoiditis
- • Neurofibroma, Schwannoma

## Treatment Options

- • Acute pain control with medications and pain management
- • Physical/Occupational/Rehabilitation therapy and rehabilitation
- • If symptomatic but poor surgical candidate (symptomatic cyst recurrence remains possible):
  - – If poor surgical candidate with poor life expectancy, medical management recommended

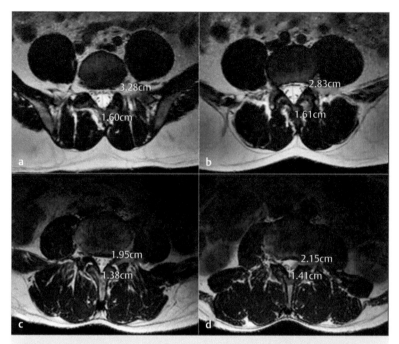

**Fig. 4.3** Cross-section images of lower lumbar Tarlov cyst patients (**a, b**) compared with normal controls (**c, d**). (Source: Xie C, Zheng X, Zhang N. Tarlov cyst is correlated with a short broad terminal of the thecal sac. J Neurol Surg A Cent Eur Neurosurg 2017;78(3):245–249).

- Lumbar drainage of CSF
- Cyst aspiration under CT guidance
- CSF removal from interior of cyst, to be injected with fibrin sealant
- If symptomatic cyst with cord/nerve root compression (treatments including, but not limited to):
  - Surgical decompression with cyst removal of implicated segments if deemed suitable candidate for surgery
    - If poor surgical candidate with poor life expectancy, medical management recommended
    - Laminectomy, cyst/nerve root removal, microsurgical cyst fenestration, and imbrication
    - Laminectomy, cyst resection

- o Microsurgical resection and defect closure with fibrin glue
- o Complete cyst removal and defect closure with fibrin glue
- o Cyst removal with neck occlusion
- If symptomatic fracture with severe central canal compression:
  - – Urgent surgical decompression and fusion of implicated segments if deemed suitable candidate for surgery
    - o If poor surgical candidate with poor life expectancy, medical management recommended
    - o Surgery may be done indirectly through axial traction or directly (posteriorly)
    - o May include a combination of the following techniques: Laminectomy (entire lamina, thickened ligaments, and part of enlarged facet joints removed to relieve pressure), Laminotomy (section of lamina and ligament removed), Foraminotomy (expanding space of neural foramen by removing soft tissues, small disk fragments, and bony spurs in the locus), Laminoplasty (expanding space within spinal canal by repositioning lamina), Diskectomy (removal of section of herniated disk), Corpectomy (removal of vertebral body and disks), Bony Spur Removal
    - o This may be accompanied by fusion for added stabilization

## Indications for Surgical Intervention

- No improvement after nonoperative therapy (physical therapy, pain management)
- Presence of radicular pain
- Neurologic dysfunction and/or instability resulting from sacral trauma or cyst

## Surgical Procedure for Posterior Sacral Spine (Cyst Excision)

1. Informed consent signed, preoperative labs normal, no Aspirin/Plavix/ Coumadin/NSAIDs/Advil/Celebrex/Ibuprofen/Motrin/Naprosyn/Aleve/ other anticoagulants and anti-inflammatory drugs for at least 2 weeks
2. Appropriate intubation and sedation and lines (if necessary) as per the anesthetist
3. Patient placed prone with all pressure points padded
4. Neuromonitoring not needed
5. Make a 5 to 7 cm incision above the appropriate level of sacral spine

6. Subperiosteally dissect paravertebral musculature until the sacral roof is exposed
7. Once the bone of interest is exposed, it is recommended to localize and verify it via X-ray or fluoroscopic imaging and confirming with at least two people in the room
8. Cut the sacral lamina at two levels, producing a bony window to expose the lateral borders of the cyst
9. Elevate the lamina off the cyst without cutting and removing it
10. Open and dissect the cyst wall with micro scissors, collapsing the cyst
11. Reinforce the occluded cyst neck using local fat graft and gelatin sponge
    a. A local muscle graft may be necessary if the cyst neck tissue is thin and its defect is large
12. Apply fibrin glue to the closure
13. Place a lumbar subarachnoid drain that can be removed in about 7 days
14. Replace the removed lamina
15. After appropriate hemostasis is obtained, muscle and skin incisions can then be closed in appropriate fashion

## Pitfalls

- Intraoperative CSF leak
- Damage to spinal nerves and/or cord (especially thecal sac injury and dural tear)
- Postoperative weakness or numbness or continued pain
- Postoperative wound infection and/or bacterial meningitis
- Continued symptoms postsurgically/unresolved symptoms with no improvement to quality of life
- Progressive kyphosis
- Problems with bowel/bladder control
- Venous thromboembolism (frequently from immobility)
- Iatrogenic nerve injury (frequently from fracture overcompression)

## Prognosis

- Hospitalization rates depend on the type of procedure performed, preoperative examination status, and patient's age/comorbidities
- Pain medications for postsurgical pain
- Physical therapy and occupational therapy will be needed postoperatively, immediately and as outpatient to regain strength
- Brace placed after discharge to immobilize to increase rate of healing

# 4.2 Elective

## 4.2.1 Sacral Decompression

### Symptoms and Signs

- Degenerate spondylolisthesis
- Diminished control/dysfunction of bladder/bowel, rectum, urinary system, and external genitalia (men: problems with erection and ejaculation; women: problems with lubrication)
- Radiculopathy of legs, buttocks, thighs, external genitalia, and perineum
- Moderate numbness in lower extremities and perianal area (saddle anesthesia)
- Paresthesia in lower body extremities
- Reduction in sensation along S2–S5
- Lower back/pelvis/thigh/buttocks pain and discomfort derived from consistent nerve irritation and loss of mobility due to the pain
- Leg pain (sciatica)
- Difficulty maintaining balance and walking
- Muscle weakness in perianal/perineal region, including difficulty in voluntarily contracting the anus
- Spinal instability

### Surgical Pathology

- Sacral spine benign/malignant trauma
- Sacral spine benign/malignant tumor
- Sacral vascular benign/malignant lesion

### Diagnostic Modalities

- Physical/Neurologic examination and patient history
- CT of sacral spine with and without contrast
- CT myelography of sacral spine
- MRI of sacral spine with and without contrast
- CT or X-ray of pelvis
- Angiography
- PET scan (search for tumor foci)
- Biopsy to examine tissue sample to determine whether tumor is benign or malignant, and what cancer type resulted in the tumor if malignancy is determined

## Differential Diagnosis

- Disk herniation(s)
- Spinal stenosis (narrowing of the spine)
- Presence of cyst or bone spurs
- Tumor:
  - Metastatic (malignant, requiring emergent treatment)
  - Primary (benign or malignant)
- Vascular lesion (typically requiring supplemental embolization):
  - Fibromuscular dysplasia (FMD)
  - Spinal arteriovenous malformation (AVM)
  - Spinal dural arteriovenous fistula (AVF)
- Vertebral trauma:
  - Zones 1–3 fractures
  - Transverse fracture
  - U-type fracture

## Treatment Options

- Acute pain control with medications and pain management
- Physical/Occupational/Rehabilitation therapy and rehabilitation
- If asymptomatic or mildly symptomatic with pain/radiculopathy with small focus of tumor:
  - Radiation treatment (radiation oncology consultation)
    ◦ Some metastatic tumors are radioresistant
  - Chemotherapy (medical oncology consultation)
    ◦ Some metastatic tumors are radioresistant
  - Kyphoplasty (to treat pain)
  - Surgical instrumentation and fusion (if there is concern for deformity, instability, or cord compression)
  - Radiosurgical intervention (if no neurologic dysfunction)
  - Sarcoplasty (if no spinal instability or neurologic dysfunction)
- If asymptomatic or mildly symptomatic trauma without neurologic injury:
  - Surgical fixation of implicated segments if deemed suitable candidate for surgery
    ◦ If poor surgical candidate with poor life expectancy, medical management recommended
    ◦ Percutaneous screw fixation
    ◦ Posterior tension band plating
    ◦ Iliosacral and lumbopelvic fixation
- If asymptomatic or mildly symptomatic with sacral cord compression:
  - Surgical decompression and fusion of implicated segments if deemed suitable candidate for surgery

- ○ If poor surgical candidate with poor life expectancy, medical management recommended
- ○ May include a combination of the following techniques: Laminectomy (entire lamina, thickened ligaments, and part of enlarged facet joints removed to relieve pressure), Laminotomy (section of lamina and ligament removed), Foraminotomy (expanding space of neural foramen by removing soft tissues, small disk fragments, and bony spurs in the locus), Laminoplasty (expanding space within spinal canal by repositioning lamina), Diskectomy (removal of section of herniated disk), Corpectomy (removal of vertebral body and disks), Bony Spur Removal, Cyst Removal
- ○ This may be accompanied by fusion for added stabilization

## Indications for Surgical Intervention

- Radicular leg pain
- Cauda equina syndrome
- No sufficient improvement of pain and symptoms after nonoperative measures (physical therapy, medications/injections, pain management)
- Sacral compression
- Significant reduction in everyday activities due to symptoms
- Expected postsurgical favorable outcome

## Sacral Procedure for Posterior Sacral Spine (Laminectomy/Foraminotomy)

1. Informed consent signed, preoperative labs normal, no Aspirin/Plavix/Coumadin/NSAIDs/Advil/Celebrex/Ibuprofen/Motrin/Naprosyn/Aleve/other anticoagulants and anti-inflammatory drugs for at least 2 weeks
2. Appropriate intubation and sedation and lines (if necessary) as per the anesthetist
3. Patient placed prone with all pressure points padded
4. Neuromonitoring not needed
5. Make a 5 to 7 cm incision above the appropriate level of sacral spine
6. Subperiosteally dissect paravertebral musculature until the sacral roof is exposed
7. Once the vertebrae of interest are exposed, it is recommended to localize and verify them via X-ray or fluoroscopic imaging and confirming with at least two people in the room
8. Perform laminectomy:
   a. Remove bilateral lamina with high-speed burr drill and Leksell rongeurs

b. Place vertical troughs bilaterally, medial to the sacral pedicles at the indicated level of spine, connected at caudal extent of laminectomy by horizontal trough

c. Extend the troughs through ventral cortex of lamina

d. Elevate lamina from underlying nerve roots using up-angled curette

e. Examine canal for nerve root injury, dural tear, and other sources of compression such as bone fragments

f. Remove such sources

9. Perform foraminotomy:

a. Dissect additional lamina, if necessary, to expose ligamentum flavum

b. Remove ligamentum flavum, thickened foraminal ligament, and bone spurs using Kerrison rongeurs with careful dissection beneath the ligament to ensure no adhesions exist to dura mater below to avoid CSF leakage

10. Perform "clean-up" as necessary:

a. Remove lingering fragments as required

b. Ablate tissue debris using a side-firing laser

11. Perform spinal fusion with instrumentation, if necessary, to ensure stability (see ▶ Fig. 4.4):

a. Place percutaneous pedicle screws over segments involved with bone grafting to fuse the indicated segments

b. Insert small drainage catheter to reduce likelihood of postoperative epidural hematoma (can be removed after 2–3 days)

12. After appropriate hemostasis is obtained, muscle and skin incisions can then be closed in appropriate fashion

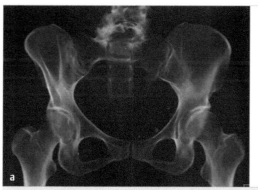
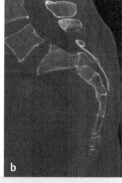

**Fig. 4.4** A patient suffering a Roy-Camille type 2 sacral fracture (**a, b**), cauda equina syndrome, kyphosis, and loss of sacral root function required realignment and decompression.

*(Continued)*

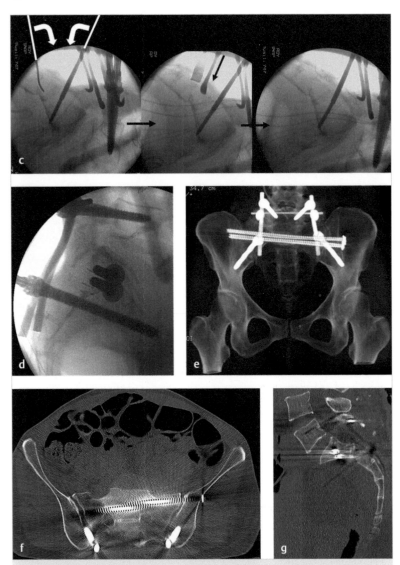

**Fig. 4.4** (*Continued*) Mobilization of the fracture was performed (**c**) to achieve proper alignment, followed by fusion with instrumentation (**d**) for stabilization. Postoperative images demonstrate adequate alignment and sacral spinal canal decompression (**e–g**). The patient's sacral root function was restored. (Source: Treatment. In: Vialle L, ed. AOSpine Masters Series, Vol. 6: Thoracolumbar Spine Trauma. 1st ed. Thieme; 2015).

## Pitfalls

- Reduction in range of motion and mobility of fused spinal segments
- Intraoperative CSF leak
- Blood clot (deep vein thrombosis, or more severe pulmonary embolism)
- Damage to spinal nerves and/or cord
- Postoperative weakness or numbness or continued pain
- Postoperative wound infection
- Prolonged hospitalization due to invasiveness of surgery and other comorbidities/iatrogenic infection
- Continued symptoms postsurgically/unresolved symptoms with no improvement to quality of life
- Loss of sensation
- Progressive kyphosis
- Residual spinal compression
- Problems with bowel/bladder control
- Recurrent disk herniation
- Vascular injury/lesions

## Prognosis

- Hospitalization rates depend on the type of procedure performed, preoperative examination status, and patient's age/comorbidities
- Pain medications for postsurgical pain
- Physical therapy and occupational therapy will be needed postoperatively, immediately and as outpatient to regain strength
- Brace placed after discharge to immobilize to increase rate of healing

# 4.2.2 Sacral Fusion

## Symptoms and Signs

- Degenerate spondylolisthesis
- Diminished control/dysfunction of bladder/bowel, rectum, urinary system, and external genitalia (men: problems with erection and ejaculation; women: problems with lubrication)
- Radiculopathy of legs, buttocks, thighs, external genitalia, and perineum
- Moderate numbness in lower extremities and perianal area (saddle anesthesia)
- Paresthesia in lower body extremities
- Reduction in sensation along S2–S5
- Lower back/pelvis/thigh/buttocks pain and discomfort derived from consistent nerve irritation and loss of mobility due to the pain

- Leg pain (sciatica)
- Difficulty maintaining balance and walking
- Muscle weakness in perianal/perineal region, including difficulty in voluntarily contracting the anus
- Spinal instability
- Pelvic ring injury
- Cauda equina symptoms

## Surgical Pathology

- Sacral spine benign/malignant trauma
- Sacral spine benign/malignant tumor
- Sacral spine benign/malignant lesion

## Diagnostic Modalities

- Physical/Neurologic examination and patient history
- CT of sacral spine with and without contrast
- CT myelography of sacral spine
- MRI of sacral spine with and without contrast
- CT or X-ray of pelvis
- Angiography
- PET scan (search for tumor foci)
- Biopsy to examine tissue sample to determine whether tumor is benign or malignant, and what cancer type resulted in the tumor if malignancy is determined

## Differential Diagnosis

- Disk herniation(s)
- Presence of cyst or bone spurs
- Tumor:
  - Metastatic (malignant, requiring emergent treatment)
  - Primary (benign or malignant)
- Vascular lesion: FMD
  - Spinal AVM
  - Spinal dural AVF
- Vertebral trauma:
  - Zones 1–3 fractures
  - Transverse fracture
  - U-type fracture

## Treatment Options

- Acute pain control with medications and pain management
- Physical/Occupational/Rehabilitation therapy and rehabilitation
  - Progressive weight bearing with or without orthosis (if no neurologic deficit and little displacement)
- If asymptomatic or mildly symptomatic with pain/radiculopathy with small focus of tumor:
  - Radiation treatment (radiation oncology consultation)
    - Some metastatic tumors are radioresistant
  - Chemotherapy (medical oncology consultation)
    - Some metastatic tumors are radioresistant
  - Kyphoplasty (to treat pain)
  - Surgical instrumentation and fusion (if concern for deformity, instability, or cord compression)
  - Radiosurgical intervention (if no neurologic dysfunction)
  - Sarcoplasty (if no spinal instability or neurologic dysfunction)
- If asymptomatic or mildly symptomatic without neurologic injury:
  - Surgical fixation of implicated segments if deemed suitable candidate for surgery:
    - If poor surgical candidate with poor life expectancy, medical management recommended with bracing
    - Percutaneous screw fixation
    - Posterior tension band plating
    - Iliosacral and lumbopelvic fixation
- If asymptomatic or mildly symptomatic with cord/nerve root compression:
  - Surgical decompression and fusion of implicated segments if deemed suitable candidate for surgery
    - If poor surgical candidate with poor life expectancy, medical management recommended
    - Surgery may be done indirectly through axial traction or directly (posteriorly)
    - May include a combination of the following techniques: Laminectomy (entire lamina, thickened ligaments, and part of enlarged facet joints removed to relieve pressure), Laminotomy (section of lamina and ligament removed), Foraminotomy (expanding space of neural foramen by removing soft tissues, small disk fragments, and bony spurs in the locus), Laminoplasty (expanding space within spinal canal by repositioning lamina), Diskectomy (removal of section of herniated disk), Corpectomy (removal of vertebral body and disks), Bony Spur Removal
    - This may be accompanied by fusion for added stabilization

## Indications for Surgical Intervention

- No sufficient improvement of pain and symptoms after nonoperative measures (physical therapy, medications/injections, pain management)
- Cauda equina syndrome
- Radicular pain
- Fracture displacement greater than 1 cm
- Fracture displacement occurs after nonoperative therapy
- Spinal instability
- Significant reduction in everyday activities due to symptoms
- Expected postsurgical favorable outcome

## Surgical Procedure for Anterior Sacral Spine (Anterior Lumbar Interbody Fusion with Transperitoneal Approach)

1. Informed consent signed, preoperative labs normal, no Aspirin/Plavix/Coumadin/NSAIDs/Advil/Celebrex/Ibuprofen/Motrin/Naprosyn/Aleve/other anticoagulants and anti-inflammatory drugs for at least 2 weeks
2. Preoperative antibiotics delivered via IV injection
3. Appropriate intubation and sedation and lines (if necessary) as per the anesthetist (endotracheal tube and ventilator-assisted breathing)
4. Patient placed in prone position on radiolucent table, enabling use of C-arm fluoroscope
5. Place sterile drapes after properly cleansing the abdominal region
6. Neuromonitoring is not needed
7. Time out is performed with agreement from everyone in the room for correct patient and correct surgery with consent signed
8. Make midline abdominal skin incision over the L5–S1 level
9. Open the linea alba by performing another midline incision
10. Spread abdominal muscles apart without cutting them
11. Retract the peritoneal sac (including the intestines) and large blood vessels to the left side using retractors
12. Visualize the anterior aspect of the intervertebral disks using retractors
13. Once the bone of interest is exposed, it is recommended to localize and verify it via fluoroscopic imaging and confirming with at least two people in the room
14. Remove the intervertebral disk using Pituitary rongeurs, Kerrison rongeurs, and curettes (diskectomy)
15. Restore normal height of disk using distractor instruments and determine the size required for cage using fluoroscopy

16. Implant metal, plastic, or bone cage (with bone graft material) into the intervertebral disk space, under fluoroscopic guidance
17. Confirm that the location is correct using fluoroscopy
18. Add stability by adding instrumentation (a plate or screws/rods to hold the cage in place) (see ▸ Fig. 4.5 and ▸ Fig. 4.6)
19. After appropriate hemostasis is obtained, muscle and skin incisions can then be closed in appropriate fashion
20. Posterior approach can then be done if further decompression needed via laminectomy, typically without need for further instrumentation and fusion
21. Standard fusion in cases without deformity is either anterior L5–S1 interbody fusion or posterior L5–S1 decompression and instrumented fusion with or without interbody graft, without need for both anterior and posterior fusion

## Pitfalls

- Reduction in range of motion and mobility of fused spinal segments
- Intraoperative CSF leak
- Urethral injury
- Bowel perforation
- Incision hernia

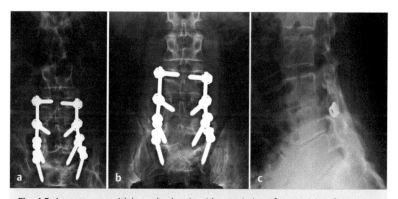

**Fig. 4.5** A young man with lower back pain without sciatica, after receiving three laminectomies, underwent alar transverse fusion at L4-Sacrum (**a**). Follow-up image (4 years) demonstrates continued stability (**b**). Solid mass of bone (L4-Sacrum) was confirmed (**c**) and his lower back pain ceased. (Source: Intertransverse fusion. In: Dickson R, Harms J, eds. Modern Management of Spinal Deformities: A Theoretical, Practical, and Evidence-based Text. 1st ed. Thieme; 2018).

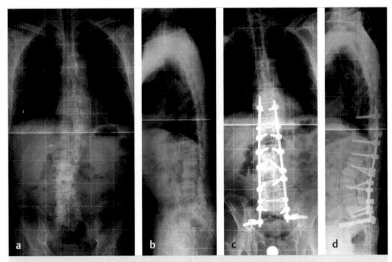

**Fig. 4.6** Radiology revealed L5–S1 degeneration (**a**) and a positive sagittal imbalance (**b**) in a middle-aged man with back pain and lumbar hypolordosis. The patient received an osteotomy at L3, followed by posterior spinal fusion at T10-Sacrum with S1 and iliac instrumentation (**c**). Postoperative sagittal balance was confirmed (**d**). (Source: Surgical decision making. In: Vialle L, ed. AOSpine Masters Series, Vol. 4: Adult Spinal Deformities. 1st ed. Thieme; 2015).

- Ileus
- Retrograde ejaculation in men
- Vascular injury
- Damage to spinal nerves and/or cord
- Postoperative weakness or numbness or continued pain
- Postoperative wound infection

## Prognosis

- Hospitalization rates depend on the type of procedure performed, preoperative examination status, and patient's age/comorbidities
- Pain medications for postsurgical pain
- Physical therapy and occupational therapy will be needed postoperatively, immediately and as outpatient to regain strength
- Brace placed after discharge to immobilize to increase rate of healing

# 4.3 Tumor/Vascular

## 4.3.1 Anterior/Posterior Sacral Tumor Resection

### Symptoms and Signs

- Radicular pain extending into legs
- Diminished control/dysfunction of bowel/bladder (including urinary retention) and external genitalia (men: problems with erection and ejaculation; women: problems with lubrication)
- Moderate/severe numbness in lower extremities and perianal area (saddle anesthesia)
- Paresthesia in lower body extremities
- Radicular pain in buttocks/thighs/legs/external genitalia/perineum
- Reduced hip mobility
- Muscle weakness in legs (paresis)
- Leg pain (sciatica)
- Difficulty maintaining balance and walking
- Local pain around tumor focus
- Local pain at sacroiliac joint(s)

### Surgical Pathology

- Sacral spine benign/malignant tumor

### Diagnostic Modalities

- Physical/Neurologic examination and patient history
- CT of sacral spine with and without contrast to assess whether there is bony involvement of tumor
- MRI of sacral spine with and without contrast to assess if there is spinal cord, epidural space, or nerve root involvement of tumor (see ▶ Fig. 4.7)
- PET scan of body to look for other foci of tumor
- CT of abdomen/pelvis to rule out metastatic disease and appendicitis
- Biopsy to examine tissue sample to determine whether tumor is benign or malignant, and what cancer type resulted in the tumor if malignancy is determined
- Endoscopic rectal examination
- Bone scan (to determine whether lesion is polyostotic)

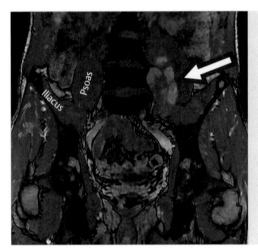

**Fig. 4.7** MRI scan revealing multifocal nerve sheath tumor. Since it extends caudally in front of the sacroiliac joint, a posterior approach to tumor resection is not ideal. A left retroperitoneal transpsoas approach is more appropriate. (Source: Transpsoas approach. In: Tubbs R, Loukas M, Hanna A, et al, eds. Surgical Anatomy of the Lumbar Plexus. 1st ed. Thieme; 2018).

## Differential Diagnosis

- Metastatic tumor
  - Breast, prostate, lung, renal cell, head/neck, gastrointestinal cell, skin (melanoma)
- Primary tumor
  - Chordoma
  - Lymphoma
  - Multiple myeloma
  - Ewing's sarcoma (in pediatrics)
  - Chondrosarcoma (in adults)
  - Osteosarcomas
- Pseudotumor
  - Giant cell tumor
  - Aneurysmal bone cyst
  - Osteoblastoma
- Paget's disease (if multiple lesions)

## Treatment Options

- Acute pain control with medications and pain management
- If asymptomatic or mildly symptomatic with lower body pain/radiculopathy with small focus of tumor:
  - Radiation treatment (radiation oncology consultation)
    - Some metastatic tumors are radioresistant

- Chemotherapy (medical oncology consultation)
  - Some metastatic tumors are radioresistant
- Kyphoplasty (to treat pain)
- Surgical instrumentation and fusion (if there is concern for deformity, instability, or cord compression)
- If symptomatic with cord compression and myelopathy with large tumor burden:
  - Urgent surgical decompression and fusion over multiple segments with tumor resection if deemed suitable candidate for surgery; may be followed by radiation treatment after resection if considered necessary by the radiation oncologist
    - Oncologist will need to determine overall prognosis, Karnofsky performance score, and extent of visceral disease
    - If poor surgical candidate with poor life expectancy, medical management recommended
    - Surgery may be done anteriorly, posteriorly, or combined two-stage approach for added stabilization (see ▸ Fig. 4.8)
  - Preoperative embolization may be indicated for select vascular tumors to the spine such as renal cell cancer, thyroid cancer, breast cancer, etc. in order to decrease vascularity intraoperatively

## Indications for Surgical Intervention

- Spinal stenosis
- No improvement after nonoperative therapy (physical therapy, pain management, radiation treatment, and chemotherapy)
- Paraplegia
- Severe canal and nerve root compression with or without myelopathy
- To obtain diagnosis if no other site for biopsy is available
- Risk of pathological fractures without stabilization

## Surgical Procedure for Anterior/Posterior Sacral Spine (En Bloc Resection)

1. Informed consent signed, preoperative labs normal, no Aspirin/Plavix/ Coumadin/NSAIDs/Advil/Celebrex/Ibuprofen/Motrin/Naprosyn/Aleve/ other anticoagulants and anti-inflammatory drugs for at least 2 weeks (see ▸ Fig. 4.9)
2. Preoperative antibiotics delivered via IV injection
3. Appropriate intubation and sedation and lines (if necessary) as per the anesthetist
4. Patient placed in supine position on radiolucent table, enabling use of C-arm fluoroscope

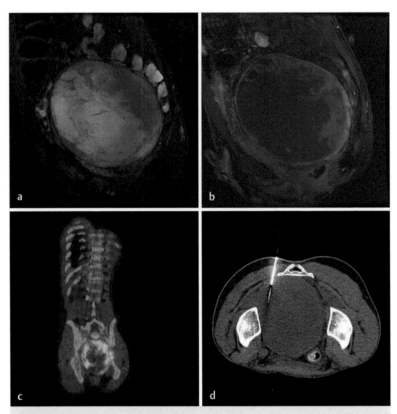

**Fig. 4.8** MRI scan of pelvis revealed a plexiform neurofibroma (**a**) in a young adult presenting with leg pain and weakness; necrosis was also visible (**b**). A PET scan revealed high avidity of tumor, characteristic of malignancies (**c**). A CT-guided needle biopsy confirmed the tumor's identity as a malignant peripheral nerve sheath tumor (**d**). (Source: Tumors of the lumbosacral plexus. In: Fessler R, Sekhar L, eds. Atlas of Neurosurgical Techniques: Spine and Peripheral Nerves. 2nd ed. Thieme; 2016).

5. Place sterile drapes after properly cleansing the abdominal region
6. Neuromonitoring not needed
7. Time out is performed with agreement from everyone in the room for correct patient and correct surgery with consent signed
8. Make incision over the rectus abdominis, exposing the internal iliac artery
9. Ligate the artery in an extraperitoneal manner and free rectum sacral space

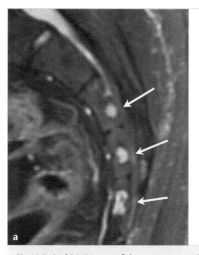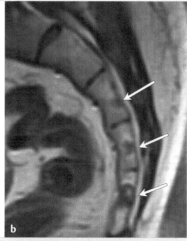

**Fig. 4.9** (a, b) MRI scan of the sacrum revealed three benign notochordal cell tumors in a middle-aged man. (Source: Lesions involving the sacrum. In: Meyers S, ed. Differential Diagnosis in Neuroimaging: Spine. 1st ed. Thieme; 2016).

10. Place large pieces of collagen sponge between ventral sacrococcyx and dorsal rectum
11. Close the anterior muscle and skin incisions in appropriate fashion
12. Transition patient into prone position
13. Make a sacral transverse incision, cutting deep fascia
14. Free the erector to expose the posterior sacral spine
15. Once the bone of interest is exposed, it is recommended to localize and verify it via fluoroscopic imaging and confirming with at least two people in the room
16. Separate attachment point of sacrum from surrounding muscles and ligaments
17. Using one finger touch the previously placed gelatin sponge through the sacrum–rectal space
18. Push the rectum to the head, separating to S2–S3 junction
19. Perform bone resection behind S2–S3 gap, exposing dural sac
20. Ligate the dural sac
    a. Resect entire S3 nerve root or leave side unmolested, on a case-by-case basis
21. Isolate the sacrum using a bone knife, removing the sacrococcygeal bone below S3

22. Flush incisions with hydrogen peroxide and diluted povidone-iodine, before immersing in distilled water
23. Leave drainage tube in left cavity
24. After appropriate hemostasis is obtained, muscle and skin incisions can then be closed in appropriate fashion
25. Then place patient prone and perform incision and identify the sacral region of interest on X-ray
26. Complete the decompression and remove sacrum with associated tumor/lesion
27. Perform hemostasis, leave drain and close in multiple layers

## Pitfalls

- Intraoperative CSF leak
- Temporary enteroplegia
- Temporary gatism
- Perianal skin hypoesthesia
- Blood clot (deep vein thrombosis, or more severe pulmonary embolism)
- Damage to spinal nerves and/or cord
- Postoperative weakness or numbness or continued pain
- Postoperative wound infection
- Continued symptoms postsurgically/unresolved symptoms with no improvement to quality of life
- Loss of sensation

## Prognosis

- Hospitalization rates depend on the type of procedure performed, preoperative examination status, and patient's age/comorbidities
- Pain medications for postsurgical pain
- Physical therapy and occupational therapy will be needed postoperatively, immediately and as outpatient to regain strength
- Back brace placed after discharge to immobilize to increase rate of healing

# Bibliography

Awad TE, Mohamed KE. Surgical excision of symptomatic sacral perineurial Tarlov cyst. Egypt J Neurosurg 2016;31(1):51–56

Elsawaf A, Awad TE, Fesal SS. Surgical excision of symptomatic sacral perineurial Tarlov cyst: case series and review of the literature. Eur Spine J 2016;25(11):3385–3392

Karadsheh M. Sacral Fractures. Orthobullets. 2018. (https://www.orthobullets.com/trauma/1032/sacral-fractures)

Mavrogenis AF, Patapis P, Kostopanagiotou G, Papagelopoulos PJ. Tumors of the sacrum. Orthopedics 2009;32(5):342

Quraishi NA, Giannoulis KE, Edwards KL, Boszczyk BM. Management of metastatic sacral tumours. Eur Spine J 2012;21(10):1984–1993

Tarlov Cyst. American Association of Neurological Surgeons. 2018. (https://www.aans. org/Patients/Neurosurgical-Conditions-and-Treatments/Tarlov-Cyst)

Tropiano P, Giorgi H, Faure A, Blondel B. Surgical techniques for lumbo-sacral fusion. Orthop Traumatol Surg Res 2017;103(1S):S151–S159

Williams SK, Quinnan SM. Percutaneous lumbopelvic fixation for reduction and stabilization of sacral fractures with spinopelvic dissociation patterns. J Orthop Trauma 2016;30(9):e318–e324

Yin X, Fan WL, Liu F, Zhu J, Liu P, Zhao JH. Technique and surgical outcome of total resection of lower sacral tumor. Int J Clin Exp Med 2015;8(2):2284–2288

# 5 Coccyx

*Christ Ordookhanian and Paul E. Kaloostian*

## 5.1 Trauma

### 5.1.1 Coccyx Fracture Repair/Resection

#### Symptoms and Signs

- Moderate/Severe pain in coccyx region (coccydynia)
- Tenderness on palpation over coccyx
- Bruising around coccyx
- Pain when moving/straining bowel
- Pain in lower back
- Radiating pain into legs

#### Surgical Pathology

- Coccyx benign/malignant trauma

#### Diagnostic Modalities

- Physical/Neurologic examination and patient history
- Rectal examination
- CT of coccyx without contrast
- MRI of coccyx without contrast
- X-ray of coccyx

#### Differential Diagnosis

- Coccyx fracture
- Coccyx fracture dislocation
- Coccyx tumor (i.e., sacrococcygeal teratoma)
- Ingrown hair cyst
- Pelvic muscle spasms
- Coccyx spicules (new bone growths)
- Referred pain from adjacent structures
  - Disk herniation(s)
  - Spinal stenosis
  - Episacral sarcoma
  - Lumbosacral lesion
  - Sacrococcygeal joint injury

## Treatment Options

- Acute pain control with medications and pain management
- Stool softeners to prevent constipation
- Coccygeal cushions
- Physical/Occupational/Recreational therapy and rehabilitation
- If symptomatic without nonsurgical improvement:
  - Urgent surgical fracture repair/resection if deemed suitable candidate for surgery
    - If poor surgical candidate with poor life expectancy, medical management recommended
    - Coccygectomy (complete removal of coccyx)
    - Removal of indicated coccygeal segments

## Indications for Surgical Intervention

- No improvement after nonoperative therapy (physical therapy, pain management, coccygeal cushion use)
- Fracture displacement after nonoperative therapy
- Unstable patterns of fracture
- Neurologic dysfunction and/or instability resulting from coccyx trauma

## Surgical Procedure for Posterior Coccyx (Coccygectomy)

1. Informed consent signed, preoperative labs normal, no Aspirin/Plavix/Coumadin/NSAIDs/Advil/Celebrex/Ibuprofen/Motrin/Naprosyn/Aleve/other anticoagulants and anti-inflammatory drugs for at least 2 weeks
2. Preoperative antibiotics are administered intravenously
3. Appropriate intubation and sedation and lines (if necessary) as per the anesthetist
4. Patient placed prone on operating table with pressure point padding
5. Neuromonitoring not needed
6. Make a 5 cm incision over the midline, 1 cm above gluteal cleft
7. Dissect past subcutaneous tissue (no muscles are present to interrupt this dissection)
8. Open fascia to expose the posterior coccyx (see ▶ Fig. 5.1)
9. Excise the intervertebral disk between the sacrum and coccyx using a scalpel
10. Bilaterally ligate/cauterize coccygeal vessels
11. Incise anococcygeal ligament and elevate tip of coccyx
12. Dissect and incise coccygeus and iliococcygeus through muscle attachments, carefully avoiding rectal injury

13. Before removing the entire coccyx, mobilize the rectum and dense fascia deep to the sacrococcygeal joint
14. Remove the entire coccyx using electrocautery
15. If tumor is present, isolate the tumor if performing en bloc coccygectomy with tumor resection or start removing tumor in piecemeal fashion

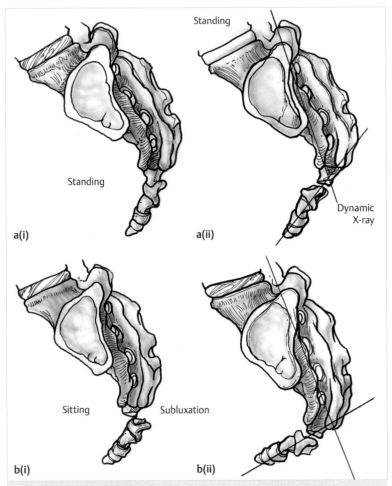

**Fig. 5.1 (a)** Illustration of sacrum and coccyx X-ray at $t = 0$ min and at $t = 10$ min. **(b)** Illustration demonstrating partial disconnection of coccyx and a high degree of flexion when sitting.

*(Continued)*

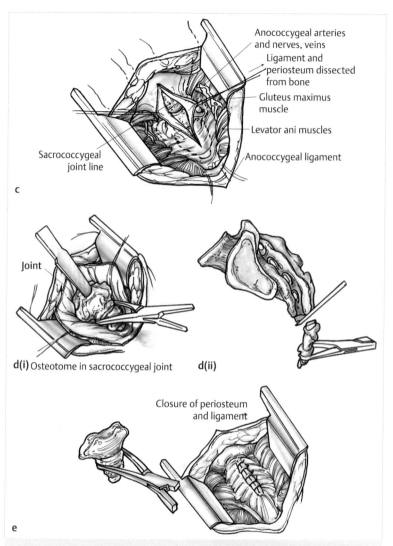

**Fig. 5.1** (*Continued*) (**c**) Illustration of exposure from terminal sacrum to painful segment of coccyx after a midline incision. (**d**) Illustration of coccygeal resection following dissection. (**e**) Illustration of excised coccyx and wound closure. (Source: Suggested readings. In: Haher T, Merola A, eds. Surgical Techniques for the Spine. 1st ed. Thieme; 2003).

16. Perform hemostasis
17. If dead space remains, place small drain
18. After appropriate hemostasis is obtained, muscle and skin incisions can then be closed in appropriate fashion

## Pitfalls

- Wound hematoma
- Postoperative weakness or numbness or continued pain
- Postoperative wound infection
- Rectal injury
- Sympathetic nerve supply injury
- Continued symptoms postsurgically/unresolved symptoms with no improvement to quality of life

## Prognosis

- Hospitalization rates depend on preoperative examination status and patient's age/comorbidities; hospitalization typically lasts about 3 days
- Pain medications for postsurgical pain
- Coccygeal cushions or other methods to reduce pain while sitting
- Physical therapy and occupational therapy will be needed postoperatively, immediately and as outpatient to regain strength
- Healing process typically lasts 3 to 12 months, depending on preoperative examination status and patient's age/comorbidities

# 5.2 Elective

## 5.2.1 Coccyx Resection

### Symptoms and Signs

- Moderate/Severe pain in coccyx region (coccydynia)
- Tenderness on palpation over coccyx
- Bruising around coccyx
- Pain when moving/straining bowel
- Pain in lower back
- Radiating pain into legs

### Surgical Pathology

- Coccyx benign/malignant trauma
- Coccyx benign/malignant tumor
- Coccyx benign/malignant cyst

## Diagnostic Modalities

- Physical/Neurologic examination and patient history
- Rectal examination (see ▶ Fig. 5.2)
- CT of coccyx without contrast
- MRI of coccyx without contrast (see ▶ Fig. 5.3)
- X-ray of coccyx
- PET scan (search for tumor foci)
- Biopsy to examine tissue sample to determine whether tumor is benign or malignant, and what cancer type resulted in the tumor if malignancy is determined

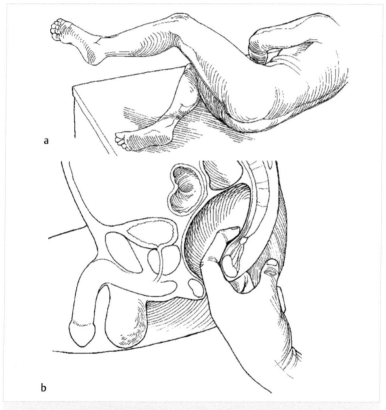

**Fig. 5.2** Illustration of patient in lateral decubitus position (**a**) in preparation for coccygeal palpation, which can be supplement testing for sphincter tone and sacral roots during rectal examination (**b**). (Source: Posterior lumbar, sacral, and coccygeal spine. In: Albert T, Vaccaro A, eds. Physical Examination of the Spine. 1st ed. Thieme; 2004).

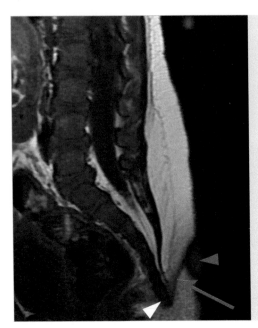

**Fig. 5.3** MRI scan of an infant demonstrating pilonidal tract (long red arrow) leading into retroflexed coccyx (white arrowhead). The red arrowhead represents the sacral dimple. (Source: Sacral dimples. In: Choudhri A, ed. Pediatric Neuroradiology: Clinical Practice Essentials. 1st ed. Thieme; 2016).

## Differential Diagnosis

- Coccyx fracture
- Coccyx fracture dislocation
- Coccyx tumor (i.e., sacrococcygeal teratoma)
- Ingrown hair cyst
- Pelvic muscle spasms
- Coccyx spicules (new bone growths)
- Referred pain from adjacent structures
  - Disk herniation(s)
  - Spinal stenosis
  - Episacral sarcoma
  - Lumbosacral lesion
  - Sacrococcygeal joint injury

## Treatment Options

- Acute pain control with medications and pain management
- Stool softeners to prevent constipation

- Coccygeal cushions
- Physical/Occupational/Recreational therapy and rehabilitation
- If asymptomatic or mildly symptomatic with pain/radiculopathy with small focus of tumor:
  - Radiation treatment (radiation oncology consultation)
    - Some metastatic tumors are radioresistant
  - Chemotherapy (medical oncology consultation)
    - Some metastatic tumors are radioresistant
  - Kyphoplasty (to treat pain)
- If asymptomatic or mildly symptomatic without nonsurgical improvement:
  - Urgent surgical fracture repair/resection if deemed suitable candidate for surgery
    - If poor surgical candidate with poor life expectancy, medical management recommended
    - Coccygectomy (complete resection of coccyx)
    - Removal of indicated coccygeal segments

## Indications for Surgical Intervention

- No sufficient improvement of pain and symptoms after nonoperative therapeutic measures (physical therapy, pain management, coccygeal cushion use)
- Fracture displacement after nonoperative therapy
- Significant reduction in everyday activities due to symptoms
- Expected postsurgical favorable outcome

## Surgical Procedure for Posterior Coccyx (Coccygectomy)

1. Informed consent signed, preoperative labs normal, no Aspirin/Plavix/Coumadin/NSAIDs/Advil/Celebrex/Ibuprofen/Motrin/Naprosyn/Aleve/other anticoagulants and anti-inflammatory drugs for at least 2 weeks
2. Preoperative antibiotics are administered intravenously
3. Appropriate intubation and sedation and lines (if necessary) as per the anesthetist
4. Patient placed prone on operating table with pressure point padding
5. Neuromonitoring not needed
6. Make a 5 cm incision over the midline, 1 cm above gluteal cleft
7. Dissect past subcutaneous tissue (no muscles are present to interrupt this dissection)
8. Open fascia to expose the posterior coccyx

9. Excise the intervertebral disk between the sacrum and coccyx using a scalpel
10. Bilaterally ligate/cauterize coccygeal vessels
11. Incise anococcygeal ligament and elevate tip of coccyx
12. Dissect and incise coccygeus and iliococcygeus through muscle attachments, carefully avoiding rectal injury
13. Before removing the entire coccyx, mobilize the rectum and dense fascia deep to the sacrococcygeal joint
14. Remove the entire coccyx using electrocautery
15. If dead space remains, place small drain
16. After appropriate hemostasis is obtained, muscle and skin incisions can then be closed in appropriate fashion

## Pitfalls

- Wound hematoma
- Postoperative weakness or numbness or continued pain
- Postoperative wound infection
- Rectal injury
- Sympathetic nerve supply injury
- Continued symptoms postsurgically/unresolved symptoms with no improvement to quality of life

## Prognosis

- Hospitalization rates depend on preoperative examination status and patient's age/comorbidities; hospitalization typically lasts about 3 to 5 days
- Pain medications for postsurgical pain
- Coccygeal cushions or other methods to reduce pain while sitting
- Physical therapy and occupational therapy will be needed postoperatively,immediately and as outpatient to regain strength
- Healing process typically lasts 3 to 12 months, depending on preoperative examination status and patient's age/comorbidities

# Bibliography

Antoniadis A, Ulrich NH, Senyurt H. Coccygectomy as a surgical option in the treatment of chronic traumatic coccygodynia: a single-center experience and literature review. Asian Spine J 2014;8(6):705–710

Gardner RC. An improved technic of coccygectomy. Clin Orthop Relat Res 1972;85 (85):143–145

# Section II

## Radiosurgery/ CyberKnife Treatment

# 6 Spinal Radiosurgery

*Ryan F. Amidon, Christ Ordookhanian, and Paul E. Kaloostian*

## 6.1 Symptoms and Signs (Broad)

- Incidental with symptoms (depending on size and location)
- Moderate/Severe numbness to pain, cold, and heat in upper or lower extremities
- Moderate/Severe back pain
- Paresthesia in upper body or lower body extremities
- Neck/Lower back/hip/lower abdominal/pelvis/buttocks pain and loss of mobility due to the pain
- Radiating pain down the arms or radicular pain extending into legs/ buttocks/thighs/external genitalia/perineum
- Pain in moving shoulders
- Muscle weakness in arms or legs (paresis) and potentially paralysis
- Inability to conduct fine motor skills with hands
- Paraplegia (partial or complete)
- Difficulty maintaining balance and walking
- Diminished control/dysfunction of bowel/bladder (including urinary retention) and external genitalia (men: problems with erection and ejaculation; women: problems with lubrication)

## 6.2 Surgical Pathology

- Spine benign/malignant tumor

## 6.3 Diagnostic Modalities

- CT of spine with and without contrast to assess whether there is bony involvement of tumor
- MRI of spine with and without contrast to assess if there is spinal cord, epidural space, or nerve root involvement of tumor
- PET scan of body to look for other foci of tumor
- CT of chest/abdomen/pelvis to rule out metastatic disease and appendicitis
- Biopsy to examine tissue sample to determine whether tumor is benign or malignant, and what cancer type resulted in the tumor if malignancy is determined

# 6.4 Differential Diagnosis

- Metastatic tumor
  - Breast, prostate, lung, renal cell
- Primary tumor
  - Intramedullary (typically reside in cervical or thoracic)
    - Astrocytoma
    - Ependymoma
    - Hemangioblastoma
    - Lipoma
  - Intradural extramedullary
    - Meningioma
    - Schwannoma
    - Neurofibroma
    - Ependymoma
  - Extradural (may reside within intervertebral foramen)

# 6.5 Treatment Options

- Acute pain control with medications and pain management
- If asymptomatic or mildly symptomatic with pain/radiculopathy with small focus of tumor:
  - Radiation treatment (radiation oncology consultation)
    - Some metastatic tumors are radioresistant
  - Chemotherapy (medical oncology consultation)
    - Some metastatic tumors are radioresistant
  - Kyphoplasty (to treat pain)
  - Surgical instrumentation and fusion (if there is concern for deformity, instability, or cord compression)
- If symptomatic with cord compression and myelopathy with large tumor burden:
  - Urgent surgical decompression and fusion of multiple segments with tumor resection if deemed suitable candidate for surgery; may be followed by radiation treatment after resection if considered necessary by the radiation oncologist
    - Oncologist will need to determine overall prognosis, Karnofsky performance score, and extent of visceral disease
    - If poor surgical candidate with poor life expectancy, medical management recommended
    - Surgery may be done anteriorly, posteriorly, or combined two-stage approach for added stabilization

- Preoperative embolization may be indicated for select vascular tumors to the spine such as renal cell cancer and thyroid cancer, breast cancer in order to decrease vascularity intraoperatively
- Radiosurgery/CyberKnife treatment (primary treatment for metastases):
  ○ The CyberKnife system includes 6-MV compact linear accelerator, two diagonal X-ray cameras, a robotic manipulator, an image detector, a treatment couch, and a treatment planning computer
  ○ A fractionated approach (small daily doses given over several weeks) may be used

## 6.6 Indications for Surgical Intervention

- No improvement after nonoperative therapy (physical therapy, pain management, radiation treatment, and chemotherapy)
- Cord compression with or without myelopathy (no indication for radiation unless myeloma)
- Metastases
- Tumor recurrence following other treatments
- Residual tumor(s) present after surgery

## 6.7 Noninvasive CyberKnife Procedure for Posterior Spine

1. Informed consent signed, preoperative labs normal
2. Place six gold seed fiducials percutaneously into posterior element of vertebrae adjacent to lesion, under fluoroscopic guidance, 1 week prior to treatment
3. Perform CT scan of 1.5 mm slice 1 day preceding treatment, using vacuum foam body cradle (see ▶ Fig. 6.1)
4. Contour the lesion and critical structures (including spine) on axial CT slices (see ▶ Fig. 6.2)
   a. This will be used to generate a three-dimensional reconstruction for the CyberKnife planning software
5. Determine treatment dose and fractionation number, considering the shape of tumor and distribution of radiation throughout the spine
6. Radiation oncologist monitors procedure
7. Place patient in supine position on CyberKnife treatment couch with appropriate immobilization (no anesthesia required)
8. Obtain X-ray images of previously implanted fiducial markers during treatment to identify location of vertebral body being treated and subsequently the tumor(s)

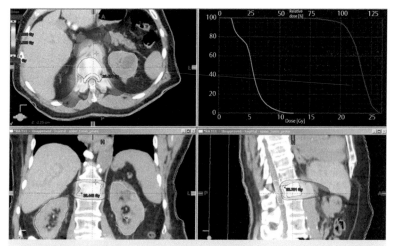

**Fig. 6.1** Spinal radiosurgery imaging setup at high-intensity (for procedures lasting less than 16 minutes) and before-and-after cone beam CT. (Source: Edge radiosurgery system for spine radiosurgery. In: Gerszten P, Ryu S, eds. Spine Radiosurgery. 2nd ed. Thieme; 2015).

9. CyberKnife robotic arm will deliver 100 to 150 nonisocentric beams sequentially, intersecting points to the tumor(s) to eliminate them via radiation (treatment lasts 30–90 minutes)
10. Number of treatments depends on the tumor size, location, and shape (one to five daily sessions typical)
11. Patients typically undergo immediate recovery due to noninvasiveness of this procedure

# 6.8 Pitfalls

- Recurrence of tumor(s) after radiosurgery due to less than optimal dosing
- Vertebral compression fracture/instability induced by radiation
- Radiation myelopathy
- Pain flare
- Esophageal toxicity
- Great vessel damage (i.e., aorta complications)

# 6.9 Prognosis

- Hospitalization is not likely, but hospitalization rates depend on the type of procedure performed, preoperative examination status, and patient's age/comorbidities

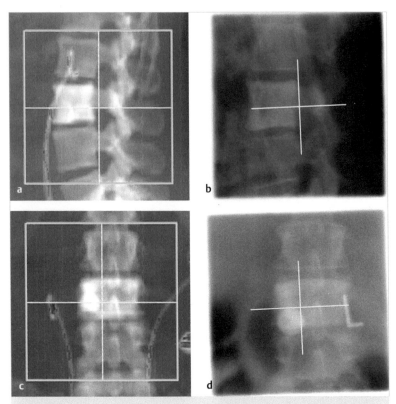

**Fig. 6.2 (a–d)** Acquire anteroposterior and lateral films and compare them with digitally reconstructed radiographs before commencing radiosurgery procedure. (Source: Quality assurance of target localization. In: Gerszten P, Ryu S, eds. Spine Radiosurgery. 1st ed. Thieme; 2015).

- MRI scan and a follow-up appointment will be scheduled with neurosurgeon or radiation oncologist
- Pain medications

# Bibliography

Chang UK, Youn SM, Park SQ, Rhee CH. Clinical results of cyberknife(r) radiosurgery for spinal metastases. J Korean Neurosurg Soc 2009;46(6):538–544

Cyberknife. UCSF Health. (https://www.ucsfhealth.org/treatments/cyberknife/)

Huo M, Sahgal A, Pryor D, Redmond K, Lo S, Foote M. Stereotactic spine radiosurgery: review of safety and efficacy with respect to dose and fractionation. Surg Neurol Int 2017;8:30

# 7 Cranial Radiosurgery

*Ryan F. Amidon, Christ Ordookhanian, and Paul E. Kaloostian*

## 7.1 Symptoms and Signs (Broad)

- Incidental with symptoms (depending on size and location)
- Headaches progressively increasing in frequency and severity
- Nausea and/or vomiting
- Blurred vision, double vision, or loss of peripheral vision
- Difficulty maintaining balance
- Reduction in sensation or motor control of certain extremities
- Difficulty producing speech
- Changes in behavior/reduction in awareness
- Seizures
- Reduction in hearing capabilities

## 7.2 Surgical Pathology

- Intracranial benign/malignant tumor
- Vascular malformation

## 7.3 Diagnostic Modalities

- Physical examination
- Neurological examination
- Cerebral angiography
- Diffusion tensor imaging (DTI)
- Single-photon emission computed tomography (SPECT) of brain
- MRI of brain
- PET scan of brain
- Optical in vivo imaging (involving bioluminescence and fluorescence)
- Biopsy of tissue

## 7.4 Differential Diagnosis

- Vascular malformation
  - Arteriovenous malformation (AVM)
- Metastatic tumor
  - Breast, colon, lung, melanoma, renal cell
- Primary tumor (may become metastatic)
  - Glioma
    - Astrocytoma (astrocytomas, anaplastic astrocytomas, glioblastomas)

- o Oligodendroglial
- o Mixed glioma (both astrocytic and oligodenrocytic)
- – Meningioma
  - o Grade I (slow growth, distinct borders)
  - o Grade II (atypical)
  - o Grade III (malignant/cancerous)
- – Schwannoma (i.e., vestibular)
- – Craniopharyngioma
- – Pituitary
- – Primary lymphoma
- – Choroid plexus papilloma/carcinoma
- – Dermoid tumor
- – Hemangioblastoma
- – Posterior fossa tumor
  - o Medulloblastoma
  - o Pineoblastoma
  - o Ependymoma
  - o Primitive neuroectodermal tumor (PNET)

# 7.5 Treatment Options

- Acute pain control with medications and pain management
- If arteriovenous malformation (AVM):
  - – Embolization to reduce AVM nidus, followed by radiosurgery
- If tumor is metastatic:
  - – Tumor resection surgery (if located in a single area of the brain) followed by radiation therapy
  - – Radiation therapy (i.e., whole-brain radiation therapy, WBRT)
  - – Immunotherapy (i.e., Yervoy, Opdivo, Keytruda)
  - – Intracranial chemotherapy or catheter-mediated chemotherapy (for leptomeningeal metastases); radiation therapy may also be used
  - – Targeted therapy
    - o Tagrisso for non-small cell lung cancer (NSCLC) with genetic alteration to EGFR gene
    - o Alecensa for NSCLC with genetic alteration to ALK gene
    - o Tykerb for HER2-positive breast cancer
    - o Tafinlar and/or Mekinist and Zelboraf for melanoma
- If tumor is deemed low grade and can be fully removed in one step (tumor is focused in one area):
  - – Tumor resection surgery
    - o Radiation therapy may be required if tumor cannot be fully removed

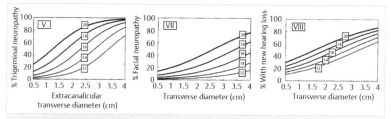

**Fig. 7.1** Graphs demonstrating relationships of extracranial tumor diameter, radiosurgery dose, and postradiation neuropathy. (Source: Introduction. In: Carlson M, Link M, Driscoll C, et al, eds. Comprehensive Management of Vestibular Schwannoma. 1st ed. Thieme; 2019).

- If tumor is deemed high grade and cannot be fully removed by surgery:
  - Tumor resection surgery if deemed suitable candidate for surgery; may be followed by radiation treatment and chemotherapy (may be supplemented by target therapy) after resection if considered necessary by the radiation oncologist
    - Oncologist will need to determine overall prognosis, Karnofsky performance score, and extent of visceral disease
    - If poor surgical candidate with poor life expectancy, medical management recommended
  - Radiation therapy:
    - Conventional radiation therapy
    - Three-dimensional conformal radiation therapy (3D-CRT)
    - Intensity modulated radiation therapy (IMRT)
    - Proton therapy
    - Radiosurgery/CyberKnife treatment (primary treatment for metastases) (see ▶ Fig. 7.1):
      - The CyberKnife system includes 6-MV compact linear accelerator, two diagonal X-ray cameras, a robotic manipulator, an image detector, a treatment couch, and a treatment planning computer
      - A fractionated approach (small daily doses given over several weeks) may be used

# 7.6 Indications for Radiosurgical Intervention

- No improvement after nonoperative therapy (physical therapy, pain management, radiation treatment, and chemotherapy)
- Metastases or primary tumor present
- Vascular malformation present
- Tumor recurrence following other treatments
- Residual tumor(s) present after surgery

# 7.7 Noninvasive CyberKnife Procedure for Cranium

1. Informed consent signed, preoperative labs normal
2. Place fiducial marker in or near tumor(s), under fluoroscopic guidance, 1 week prior to treatment
3. Prior to treatment:
   a. Cover patient's face/head with fitted mesh mask (no stereotactic head frames needed for CyberKnife treatment)
   b. Perform CT or MRI to confirm location of tumor(s)
      i. AVM identification utilizes CT, MRI, and/or cerebral angiograms
      ii. Trigeminal neuralgia imaging utilizes CT or MRI
   c. The imaging results are incorporated into the CyberKnife planning system to aid in the planning of dosage and fractionation number
   d. Radiation oncologist conducts simulation to determine optimal position of body to align with radiation beams
   e. Keep patient stable with immobilization equipment
   f. Take imaging scans to plan the optimal combination of radiation beams to target tumor(s) or other abnormalities
4. On treatment day:
   a. If nil per os, intravenous line may deliver fluids to blood stream
   b. Radiation oncologist monitors procedure
   c. Place patient in supine position on CyberKnife treatment couch with appropriate immobilization (no anesthesia required)
   d. Perform imaging of previously implanted fiducial marker during treatment to identify location of tumor(s)
   e. CyberKnife robotic arm will deliver 100 to 150 nonisocentric beams sequentially, intersecting points to the tumor(s) to eliminate them via radiation
   f. Number of treatments depends on the tumor size, location, and shape
   g. Patients typically experience immediate recovery due to noninvasiveness of this procedure

# 7.8 Pitfalls

- Recurrence of tumor(s) after radiosurgery due to less than optimal dosing
- Local brain swelling
- Scalp and hair problems
- Vision or hearing loss (see ▶ Fig. 7.2)
- Neurocognition deficits from WBRT

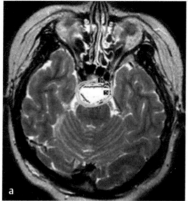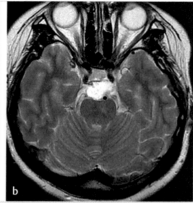

**Fig. 7.2** Gamma knife radiosurgery was employed to treat a young adult woman's chordoma (**a**). Follow-up imaging (7 years) demonstrates reduced size of tumor (**b**). (Source: Chordoma. In: Sekhar L, Fessler R, eds. Atlas of Neurosurgical Techniques: Brain, Vol. 2. 2nd ed. Thieme; 2015).

## 7.9 Prognosis

- Hospitalization is not likely, but hospitalization rates depend on the type of procedure performed, preoperative examination status, and patient's age/comorbidities
- Headache, nausea, or vomiting, if present following the procedure, will warrant relevant medications
- MRI scan and a follow-up appointment will be scheduled with neurosurgeon or radiation oncologist
- Pain medications

## Bibliography

Brain Tumor. Mayo Clinic. 2019. (https://www.mayoclinic.org/diseases-conditions/brain-tumor/symptoms-causes/syc-20350084)

Brain Tumor–Primary–Adults. MedlinePlus. 2019. (https://medlineplus.gov/ency/article/007222.htm)

Brain Tumor: Types of Treatment. Cancer.Net. 2019. (https://www.cancer.net/cancer-types/brain-tumor/types-treatment)

Cyberknife. UCSF Health. (https://www.ucsfhealth.org/treatments/cyberknife/)

Gao H, Jiang X. Progress on the diagnosis and evaluation of brain tumors. Cancer Imaging 2013;13(4):466–481

Sheehan JP, Yen CP, Lee CC, Loeffler JS. Cranial stereotactic radiosurgery: current status of the initial paradigm shifter. J Clin Oncol 2014;32(26):2836–2846

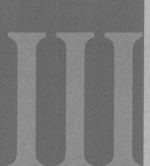

# Section III

**Cranial Lesion Resection (Brain Tumor, Vascular Lesions)**

# 8 Brain Tumors

*Ryan F. Amidon, Christ Ordookhanian, and Paul E. Kaloostian*

## 8.1 Meningioma Convexity/Olfactory Groove Meningioma

### 8.1.1 Symptoms and Signs

- Incidental with symptoms (depending on size and location)
- Loss of smell and taste
- Blurred vision
- Memory loss
- Headaches
- Fatigue/nausea
- Vomiting
- Changes in personality
- Seizures
- Neurological deficits
- Vertigo
- Syncope/fainting
- Symptoms may not be present

### 8.1.2 Surgical Pathology

- Cranial benign/malignant tumor

### 8.1.3 Diagnostic Modalities

- Physical examination
- Neurological examination
- Cerebral angiography
- Diffusion tensor imaging (DTI)
- Single-photon emission computed tomography (SPECT) of brain
- MRI of brain (often required to find olfactory groove meningiomas since symptoms are not typically present)
- PET scan of brain
- Optical in vivo imaging (involving bioluminescence and fluorescence)
- Biopsy of tissue

## 8.1.4 Differential Diagnosis

- Metastatic tumor
  - Breast, colon, lung, melanoma, renal cell
- Primary tumor (may become metastatic)
  - Glioma
    ○ Astrocytoma (astrocytomas, anaplastic astrocytomas, glioblastomas)
    ○ Oligodendroglial
    ○ Mixed glioma (both astrocytic and oligodenrocytic)
  - Meningioma
    ○ Olfactory groove meningioma (typically benign) (see ▶ Fig. 8.1)
    ○ Convexity meningioma (notably surgically accessible) (see ▶ Fig. 8.2)
    ○ Grade I (slow growth, distinct borders)
    ○ Grade II (atypical)
    ○ Grade III (malignant/cancerous)
  - Schwannoma
  - Craniopharyngioma

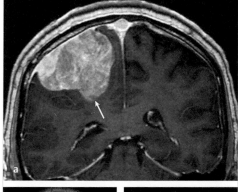

**Fig. 8.1** (a–c) MRI scans reveal malignant meningioma at right convexity. Diffusion-weighted imaging reveals restricted diffusion at meningioma locus. (Source: Introduction. In: Meyers S, ed. Differential Diagnosis in Neuroimaging: Brain and Meninges. 1st ed. Thieme; 2016).

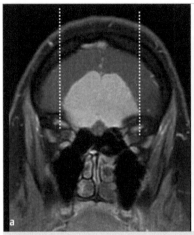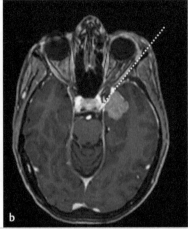

**Fig. 8.2** MRI scan reveals olfactory groove meningioma centered at the midline with confined lateral projections (**a**). Complete resection via an endonasal route is possible. (**b**) The MRI scan reveals sphenoid wing meningioma, in which case an endonasal approach is not appropriate. (Source: Expanded endonasal approaches to nonpituitary tumors. In: Nader R, Gragnaniello C, Berta S, et al, eds. Neurosurgery Tricks of the Trade: Cranial. 1st ed. Thieme; 2013).

- Pituitary
- Primary lymphoma
- Choroid plexus papilloma/carcinoma
- Dermoid tumor
- Hemangioblastoma
- Posterior fossa tumor
  - Medulloblastoma
  - Pineoblastoma
  - Ependymoma
  - Primitive neuroectodermal tumor (PNET)
  - Astrocytoma of cerebellum and brainstem

## 8.1.5 Treatment Options

- Acute pain control with medications and pain management
- If tumor is metastatic:
  - Tumor resection surgery (if located in a single area of the brain) followed by radiation therapy
  - Radiation therapy (i.e., whole-brain radiation therapy, WBRT)

- Immunotherapy (i.e., Yervoy, Opdivo, Keytruda)
- Intracranial chemotherapy or catheter-mediated chemotherapy (for leptomeningeal metastases); radiation therapy may also be used
- Targeted therapy
  ○ Tagrisso for non-small cell lung cancer (NSCLC) with genetic alteration to EGFR gene
  ○ Alecensa for NSCLC with genetic alteration to ALK gene
  ○ Tykerb for HER2-positive breast cancer
  ○ Tafinlar and/or Mekinist and Zelboraf for melanoma
- If tumor is deemed low grade and can be fully removed in one step (tumor is focused in one area):
  - Tumor resection surgery
    ○ Radiation therapy may be required if tumor cannot be fully removed
    ○ Transnasal endoscopic surgery if small and easily reachable (typically for olfactory groove meningioma)
    ○ Craniotomy or minicraniotomy approaches (removing part of the skull to resect tumor)
    ○ Pterional approach (shortest route to suprasellar cisterns)
    ○ Embolization performed prior to surgery if meningioma is large and has rich vascular supply
- If tumor is deemed high grade and cannot be fully removed by surgery:
  - Tumor resection surgery if deemed suitable candidate for surgery; may be followed by radiation treatment and chemotherapy (may be supplemented by target therapy) after resection if considered necessary by the radiation oncologist
    ○ Oncologist will need to determine overall prognosis, Karnofsky performance score, and extent of visceral disease
    ○ If poor surgical candidate with poor life expectancy, medical management recommended
  - Radiation therapy
    ○ Conventional Radiation Therapy
    ○ Three-dimensional conformal radiation therapy (3D-CRT)
    ○ Intensity modulated radiation therapy (IMRT)
    ○ Proton therapy
    ○ Radiosurgery/CyberKnife treatment (primary treatment for metastases)

## 8.1.6 Indications for Surgical Intervention

- No improvement after nonoperative therapy (physical therapy, pain management, radiation treatment, and chemotherapy)
- Metastasis in single brain location

- Large tumor(s) causing significant mass effect or obstructive hydrocephalus
- Patient does not possess more than four brain lesions from multiple metastases
- Tumor(s) surgically accessible
- Tumor recurrence following other treatments
- Residual tumor(s) present after surgery

## 8.1.7 Surgical Procedure for Bifrontal Craniotomy (Pre-op Embolization Can Be Done Prior to Surgery)

1. Informed consent signed, preoperative labs normal, patient ceases intaking of NSAIDs (Naprosyn, Advil, Nuprin, Motrin, Aleve) and blood thinners (Coumadin, Plavix, Aspirin) 1 week prior to treatment
2. Maintain patients with preoperative seizures on antiepileptic for 1 year
3. Patient's head is shaved and skin overlaying surgical site is cleansed with antiseptic solution
4. Appropriate intubation and sedation and lines (if necessary) as per the anesthetist
5. Intravenously administer 1 g third-generation cephalosporin antibiotic, 10 mg dexamethasone, 1 g phenytoin
6. Place patient in supine position on operating table, with Mayfield Pin fixation and minor head extension, and all pressure points padded
7. Neuromonitoring not needed
8. Time out is performed with agreement from everyone in the room for correct patient and correct surgery with consent signed
9. Incise skin from zygoma to zygoma, within 1 cm of tragus (avoiding injury to superficial temporal artery)
10. Turn skin flap and administer 200 mL mannitol
11. Open the dura and raise pericranium and its pedicle of blood vessels, to be used in reconstruction of anterior skull base
12. Place two burr holes bilaterally at keyholes on frontosphenoid suture, 6 mm posterior to frontozygomatic suture
13. Place one burr hole on each side of sagittal sinus in midline (to straddle sinus)
14. Release sinus dura from undersurface of bone using blunt Penfield dissector
15. Complete craniotomy using craniotome, incorporating frontal sinus flushed with anterior cranial base
16. Cranialize frontal sinuses by removing its mucosa and posterior wall

17. Remove crista galli
18. Perform dural coagulation on dural vessels
19. Bring microscope into operating field for use in remaining steps
20. Elevate dura from anterior cranial base and devascularize extradural tumor
21. Coagulate anterior and posterior ethmoidal arteries
22. Open dura in straight line along frontal poles
23. Suture sagittal sinus and cut along falx, just above the crista galli
24. Retract frontal lobes to approach tumor (facilitated by draining cerebrospinal fluid [CSF] from nearby cisterns), using suction tip
25. Perform extracapsular coagulation and internal debulking
26. Move capsule toward center and develop a plane between capsule and surrounding brain
27. Meningiomas are situated in subdural space outside the arachnoid
28. Remove tumor from anterior to posterior until optic apparatus and anterior cerebral arteries and branches are visible
29. Carefully separate tumor capsule from this structure
30. If tumor invades into optic canal, remove it by sectioning falciform ligament and decompressing optic nerve
31. If tumor invades into upper half of ethmoid sinuses, remove it by entering ethmoid sinuses from above, angling microscope into the sinus, releasing slightly more CSF from lumbar drain with minimal retraction applied to frontal lobe
32. Reconstruct anterior cranial base
    a. Vascularized pericranium previously raised as a separate layer during procedure is reflected inferiorly in wet gauze
    b. After tumor removal and drilling the hyperostotic bone, lay vascularized pericranium over base of anterior cranial base
    c. Apply two stitches on each side of base of anterior fossa
    d. Place subgaleal drain if deemed necessary
    e. Close dura in standard fashion
    f. Close galea and skin in standard fashion

## 8.1.8 Pitfalls

- Neurologic deficits
- Vascular injury during tumor resection
- Frontal lobe retraction-related injury
- Olfactory loss
- Postoperative seizure
- Reduction in visual acuity

## 8.1.9 Prognosis

- Patient will be taken to a recovery room and ultimately to the intensive care unit (ICU). Hospitalization rates depend on the type of procedure performed, preoperative examination status, and patient's age/comorbidities (discharge after 2–7 days typical).
- Patient will have to enroll in rehabilitation unit for several days after hospital stay
- Patient will have sequential compression devices (SCDs) placed on legs while in bed to reduce chance of blood clot formation
- Headache, nausea, or vomiting, if present following the procedure, will warrant relevant medications
- Abstain from heavy lifting for 2 weeks
- Patients without preoperative seizures are placed on antiepileptic for 1 week postoperatively

# 8.2 Metastatic Tumor Resection

## 8.2.1 Symptoms and Signs (Broad)

- Incidental with symptoms (depending on size and location)
- Headaches progressively increasing in frequency and severity
- Nausea and/or vomiting
- Blurred vision, double vision, or loss of peripheral vision
- Difficulty maintaining balance
- Reduction in sensation or motor control of certain extremities
- Difficulty producing speech
- Changes in behavior/reduction in awareness
- Seizures
- Reduction in hearing capabilities

## 8.2.2 Surgical Pathology

- Cranial benign/malignant tumor

## 8.2.3 Diagnostic Modalities

- Physical examination
- Neurological examination
- Cerebral angiography DTI
- SPECT of brain
- MRI of brain (see ▶ Fig. 8.3 and ▶ Fig. 8.4)

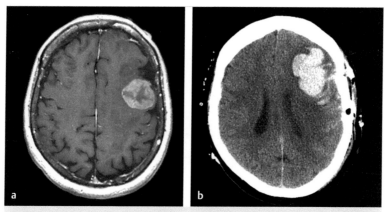

**Fig. 8.3** MRI scan revealed a left frontal metastatic tumor in middle-aged woman with a history of breast cancer presenting with generalized seizure (**a**). She received tumor resection and a follow-up CT scan (1 day) revealed significant hemorrhage in resection cavity (**b**). The hematoma was evacuated and full recovery was achieved. (Source: Surgical complications and their avoidance. In: Bernstein M, Berger M, eds. Neuro-Oncology: The Essentials. 3rd ed. Thieme; 2014).

- PET scan of brain
- Optical in vivo imaging (involving bioluminescence and fluorescence)
- Biopsy of tissue

## 8.2.4 Differential Diagnosis

- Metastatic tumor
  - Breast, colon, lung, melanoma, renal cell
- Primary tumor (may become metastatic)
  - Glioma
    - ◦ Astrocytoma (astrocytomas, anaplastic astrocytomas, glioblastomas)
    - ◦ Oligodendroglial
      Mixed glioma (both astrocytic and oligodenrocytic)
  - Meningioma
    - ◦ Grade I (slow growth, distinct borders)
    - ◦ Grade II (atypical)
    - ◦ Grade III (malignant/cancerous)
  - Schwannoma
  - Craniopharyngioma
  - Pituitary

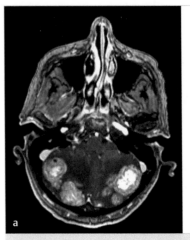 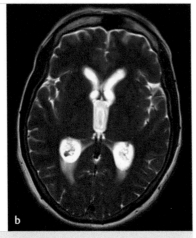

**Fig. 8.4 (a, b)** Radiology revealed hydrocephalus from metastasis reaching posterior fossa in middle-aged woman with a history of breast cancer presenting with headache and vomiting. She received a ventriculoperitoneal shunt and recovery was achieved (Source: Epidemiology, clinical presentation, and pathogenesis. In: Albright A, Pollack I, Adelson P, eds. Principles and Practice of Pediatric Neurosurgery. 3rd ed. Thieme; 2014).

- Primary lymphoma
- Choroid plexus papilloma/carcinoma
- Dermoid tumor
- Hemangioblastoma
- Posterior fossa tumor (see ▶ Fig. 8.5 and ▶ Fig. 8.6)
  - Medulloblastoma
  - Pineoblastoma
  - Ependymoma
  - PNET
  - Astrocytoma of cerebellum and brainstem

## 8.2.5 Treatment Options

- Acute pain control with medications and pain management
- If tumor is metastatic:
  - Tumor resection surgery (if located in a single area of the brain) followed by radiation therapy
  - Radiation therapy (i.e., WBRT)
  - Immunotherapy (i.e., Yervoy, Opdivo, Keytruda)

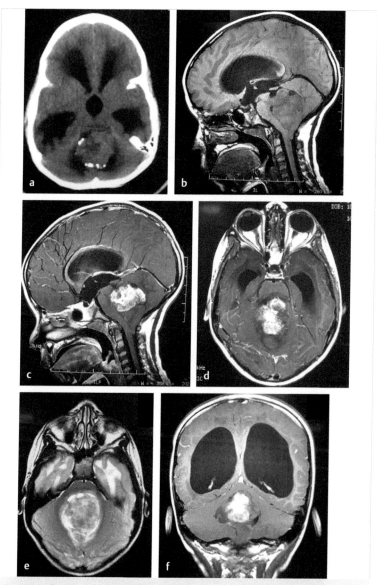

**Fig. 8.5** (a–f) MRI scan reveals posterior fossa tumor and associated hydrocephalus in a 7-year-old boy. A cerebellar pilocytic astrocytoma variety was identified and a suboccipital craniotomy was performed. (Source: Astrocytic tumors. In: Bernstein M, Berger M, eds. Neuro-Oncology: The Essentials. 3rd ed. Thieme; 2014).

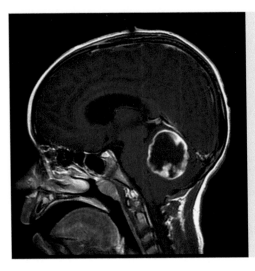

**Fig. 8.6** MRI (FLAIR) demonstrating pituitary tumor and its carotid encasement and suprasellar extension. (Source: Preoperative considerations. In: Stamm A, ed. Transnasal Endoscopic Skull Base and Brain Surgery: Surgical Anatomy and Its Applications. 2nd ed. Thieme; 2019).

- Intracranial chemotherapy or catheter-mediated chemotherapy (for leptomeningeal metastases); radiation therapy may also be used
- Targeted therapy
  - Tagrisso for NSCLC with genetic alteration to EGFR gene
  - Alecensa for NSCLC with genetic alteration to ALK gene
  - Tykerb for HER2-positive breast cancer
  - Tafinlar and/or Mekinist and Zelboraf for melanoma
- If tumor is deemed low grade and can be fully removed in one step (tumor is focused in one area):
  - Tumor resection surgery
    - Radiation therapy may be required if tumor cannot be fully removed
    - Transnasal endoscopic surgery if small and easily reachable (typically for olfactory groove meningioma)
    - Craniotomy or minicraniotomy approaches (removing part of the skull to resect tumor)
    - Pterional approach (shortest route to suprasellar cisterns)
    - Embolization performed prior to surgery if meningioma is large and has rich vascular supply
- If tumor is deemed high grade and cannot be fully removed by surgery:
  - Tumor resection surgery if deemed suitable candidate for surgery; may be followed by radiation treatment and chemotherapy (may be supplemented by target therapy) after resection if considered necessary by the radiation oncologist

- Oncologist will need to determine overall prognosis, Karnofsky performance score, and extent of visceral disease
- If poor surgical candidate with poor life expectancy, medical management recommended
  - Radiation therapy
    - Conventional radiation therapy
    - 3D-CRT
    - IMRT
    - Proton therapy
    - Radiosurgery/CyberKnife treatment (primary treatment for metastases)

## 8.2.6 Indications for Surgical Intervention

- No improvement after nonoperative therapy (physical therapy, pain management, radiation treatment, and chemotherapy)
- Metastasis in single brain location
- Large tumor(s) of over 3 cm causing significant mass effect or obstructive hydrocephalus
- Patient does not possess more than four brain lesions from multiple metastases
- Tumor(s) surgically accessible
- Tumor recurrence following other treatments
- Residual tumor(s) present after surgery

## 8.2.7 Surgical Procedure for Craniotomy

1. Informed consent signed, preoperative labs normal, patient ceases intaking of NSAIDs (Naprosyn, Advil, Nuprin, Motrin, Aleve) and blood thinners (Coumadin, Plavix, Aspirin) 1 week prior to treatment
2. Appropriate intubation and sedation and lines (if necessary) as per the anesthetist
3. Intravenously administer 1 g third-generation cephalosporin antibiotic, 10 mg dexamethasone
4. Patient's head is shaved and skin overlaying surgical site is cleansed with antiseptic solution
5. Place patient in a position appropriate for reaching the tumor location on operating table, with Mayfield Pin fixation, and all pressure points padded
6. Neuromonitoring not needed
7. Time out is performed with agreement from everyone in the room for correct patient and correct surgery with consent signed
8. Incise skin in location appropriate for reaching the location of tumor

9. Pull the scalp up and clip it to control bleeding, allowing access to brain
10. Make burr holes in the skull using a medical drill and carefully cut the bone using a saw, if necessary
11. Remove the bone flap, saving it for future steps
12. Separate the dura mater from the bone and cut it, exposing the brain
13. Microsurgical instruments may be utilized to better distinguish abnormal and healthy tissues in relevant brain structures
14. Ensure that all surgically accessible tumor components have been resected and that hemostasis has been achieved
15. Suture the dura mater
16. Reattach the bone flap using plates, sutures, or wires
    a. If a tumor or infection is present in the bone, do not reattach it
    b. If decompression is required, do not reattach the bone flap
17. Close skin incision with sutures or surgical staples
18. Apply sterile bandage or dressing over incision

## 8.2.8 Pitfalls

- Recurrence of tumor(s) after surgery
- Neurologic deficits
- Vascular injury during tumor resection
- Blood clots
- Pneumonia
- Seizures
- Brain swelling
- CSF leakage
- Paralysis, memory deficits, difficulty producing speech, diminished balance, and/or coma (rare)

## 8.2.9 Prognosis

- Patient will be taken to a recovery room and ultimately to the ICU. Hospitalization rates depend on the type of procedure performed, preoperative examination status, and patient's age/comorbidities (discharge after 3–7 days typical).
- Patient will have to enroll in rehabilitation unit for several days after hospital stay
- Patient will have SCDs placed on legs while in bed to reduce chance of blood clot formation
- Headache, nausea, or vomiting, if present following the procedure, will warrant relevant medications

# 8.3 Posterior Fossa Tumor Resection

## 8.3.1 Symptoms and Signs

- Incidental with symptoms (depending on size and location)
- Headaches progressively increasing in frequency and severity
- Nausea, drowsiness, and/or vomiting
- Difficulty maintaining balance, diminishing motor control and coordination
- Ataxia
- Hydrocephalus
- Strabismus
- Blurred vision
- Meningismus
- Apnea
- Macrocephaly (children)

## 8.3.2 Surgical Pathology

- Cranial benign/malignant tumor

## 8.3.3 Diagnostic Modalities

- Physical examination
- Neurological examination
- Cerebral angiography DTI
- SPECT of brain
- MRI of brain
- PET scan of brain
- Optical in vivo imaging (involving bioluminescence and fluorescence)
- Biopsy of tissue

## 8.3.4 Differential Diagnosis

- Metastatic tumor
  - Breast, colon, lung, melanoma, renal cell
- Primary tumor (may become metastatic)
  - Glioma
    - Astrocytoma (astrocytomas, anaplastic astrocytomas, glioblastomas)
    - Oligodendroglial
    - Mixed glioma (both astrocytic and oligodenrocytic)

- Meningioma
  - Grade I (slow growth, distinct borders)
  - Grade II (atypical)
  - Grade III (malignant/cancerous)
- Schwannoma
- Craniopharyngioma
- Pituitary
- Primary lymphoma
- Choroid plexus papilloma/carcinoma
- Dermoid tumor
- Hemangioblastoma
- Posterior fossa tumor
  - Medulloblastoma
  - Pineoblastoma
  - Ependymoma
  - PNET
  - Cerebellar astrocytoma

## 8.3.5 Treatment Options

- Acute pain control with medications and pain management
- If tumor is metastatic:
  - Tumor resection surgery (if located in a single area of the brain) followed by radiation therapy
  - Radiation therapy (i.e., WBRT)
  - Immunotherapy (i.e., Yervoy, Opdivo, Keytruda)
  - Intracranial chemotherapy or catheter-mediated chemotherapy (for leptomeningeal metastases); radiation therapy may also be used
  - Targeted therapy
    - Tagrisso for NSCLC with genetic alteration to EGFR gene
    - Alecensa for NSCLC with genetic alteration to ALK gene
    - Tykerb for HER2-positive breast cancer
    - Tafinlar and/or Mekinist and Zelboraf for melanoma
- If tumor is deemed low grade and can be fully removed in one step (tumor is focused in one area):
  - Tumor resection surgery
    - Radiation therapy may be required if tumor cannot be fully removed
    - Transnasal endoscopic surgery if small and easily reachable (typically for olfactory groove meningioma)
    - Craniotomy or minicraniotomy approaches (removing part of the skull to resect tumor)

- ○ Pterional approach (shortest route to suprasellar cisterns)
- ○ Embolization performed prior to surgery if meningioma is large and has rich vascular supply
- If tumor is deemed high grade and cannot be fully removed by surgery:
  - Tumor resection surgery if deemed suitable candidate for surgery; may be followed by radiation treatment and chemotherapy (may be supplemented by target therapy) after resection if considered necessary by the radiation oncologist
    - ○ Oncologist will need to determine overall prognosis, Karnofsky performance score, and extent of visceral disease
    - ○ If poor surgical candidate with poor life expectancy, medical management recommended
  - Radiation therapy
    - ○ Conventional radiation therapy
    - ○ 3D-CRT
    - ○ IMRT
    - ○ Proton therapy
    - ○ Radiosurgery/CyberKnife treatment (primary treatment for metastases)

## 8.3.6 Indications for Surgical Intervention

- No improvement after nonoperative therapy (physical therapy, pain management, radiation treatment, and chemotherapy)
- Large tumor of over 3 cm causing significant mass effect or obstructive hydrocephalus
- Patient does not possess more than four brain lesions from multiple metastases
- Tumor surgically accessible
- Tumor recurrence following other treatments
- Residual tumor(s) present after surgery

## 8.3.7 Surgical Procedure for Posterior Fossa Craniectomy

1. Informed consent signed, preoperative labs normal, patient ceases intaking of NSAIDs (Naprosyn, Advil, Nuprin, Motrin, Aleve) and blood thinners (Coumadin, Plavix, Aspirin) 1 week prior to treatment
2. Administer glucocorticoids (i.e., dexamethasone) in a 1 mg/kg/day dose
3. Appropriate intubation and sedation and lines (if necessary) as per the anesthetist

4. Patient's head is shaved and skin overlaying surgical site is cleansed with antiseptic solution
5. Place patient in prone position on operating table, with Mayfield Pin fixation, and all pressure points padded
6. Neuromonitoring not needed
7. Time out is performed with agreement from everyone in the room for correct patient and correct surgery with consent signed
8. Make safety burr hole in occipital area, for use in the case of acute hydrocephalus requiring ventricular drainage
   a. Patients with hydrocephalus will require =a cannula through this burr hole, with a subcutaneous catheter connected to external ventricular drainage system
9. Perform midline incision from inion to upper cervical vertebra
10. Separate paracervical and suboccipital muscles by diathermy
11. Perform craniectomy according to the site and size of tumor
12. Open foramen magnum and remove C1 arch
13. Open dura in a Y-shape, with base upward
14. Incise cerebellar cortex using bipolar and self-retaining retractors, exposing the tumor
15. Remove the tumor via gentle suction or ultrasonic surgical aspirator
16. Close dura in standard fashion
    a. Perform dural grafting if necessary
17. Control CSF circulation perioperatively using Ommaya reservoir to safely and wholly remove tumors (often not needed)
18. If choroid plexus papilloma, remove entirely
19. If dermoid cyst is associated with a sinus, remove sinus entirely
20. Reattach bone flap using plates, sutures, or wires
    a. If a tumor or infection is present in the bone, do not reattach it
    b. If decompression is required, do not reattach the bone flap
21. Close skin incision with sutures or surgical staples
22. Apply sterile bandage or dressing over incision

## 8.3.8 Pitfalls

- Infection
- Apnea
- Lower cranial nerve dysfunction
- Increased ataxia
- Facial nerve palsy

- Deafness
- Hemiplegia
- Hemiparesis
- Sensory abnormalities
- Coma
- Deep venous thrombosis
- Pulmonary embolism
- CSF leakage
- Ocular motor abnormalities
- Cerebellar mutism syndrome

## 8.3.9 Prognosis

- Patient will be taken to a recovery room and ultimately to the ICU. Hospitalization rates depend on the type of procedure performed, preoperative examination status, and patient's age/comorbidities.
- Patient will have to enroll in rehabilitation unit for several days after hospital stay
- Patient will have SCDs placed on legs while in bed to reduce chance of blood clot formation
- Headache, nausea, or vomiting, if present following the procedure, will warrant relevant medications

# 8.4 Pituitary Tumor Resection

## 8.4.1 Symptoms and Signs

- Incidental with symptoms (depending on size and location)
- Headaches progressively increasing in frequency and severity
- Nausea, drowsiness, and/or vomiting
- Personality change
- Vision abnormalities
- Cushing's syndrome
- Acromegaly
- Alterations to menstrual cycle (women)
- Abnormal production of breast milk (women)
- Erectile dysfunction (men)
- Infertility

## 8.4.2  Surgical Pathology

- Cranial benign/malignant tumor

## 8.4.3  Diagnostic Modalities

- Physical examination
- Neurological examination
- Visual field exam
- Cerebral angiography DTI
- SPECT of brain
- MRI of brain
- PET scan of brain
- Optical in vivo imaging (involving bioluminescence and fluorescence)
- Biopsy

## 8.4.4  Differential Diagnosis

- Metastatic tumor
  – Breast, colon, lung, melanoma, renal cell
- Primary tumor (may become metastatic)
  – Glioma
    ○ Astrocytoma (astrocytomas, anaplastic astrocytomas, glioblastomas)
    ○ Oligodendroglial
    ○ Mixed glioma (both astrocytic and oligodenrocytic)
  – Meningioma
    ○ Grade I (slow growth, distinct borders)
    ○ Grade II (atypical)
    ○ Grade III (malignant/cancerous)
  – Schwannoma
  – Craniopharyngioma
  – Pituitary gland (see ▶ Fig. 8.7 to ▶ Fig. 8.9)
  – Primary lymphoma
  – Choroid plexus papilloma/carcinoma
  – Dermoid tumor
  – Hemangioblastoma
  – Posterior fossa tumor
    ○ Medulloblastoma
    ○ Pineoblastoma
    ○ Ependymoma
    ○ PNET
    ○ Cerebellar astrocytoma

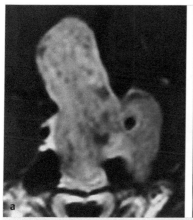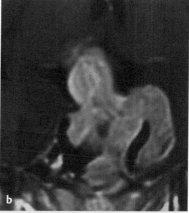

**Fig. 8.7** (**a, b**) MRI (FLAIR) demonstrating pituitary tumor and its carotid encasement and suprasellar extension. (Source: Pathology of sellar and parasellar lesions. In: Stamm A, ed. Transnasal Endoscopic Skull Base and Brain Surgery: Surgical Anatomy and Its Applications. 2nd ed. Thieme; 2019).

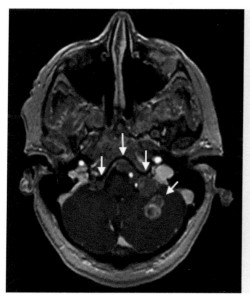

**Fig. 8.8** MRI scan reveals giant pituitary tumor elevating the diaphragma sellae. (Source: The use of the endoscope in pituitary tumor surgery. In: Al-Mefty O, ed. Controversies in Neurosurgery II. 1st ed. Thieme; 2013).

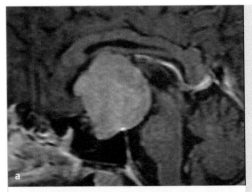

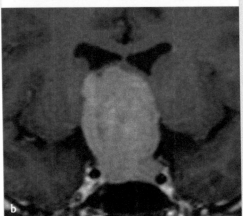

Fig. 8.9 (a, b) MRI scans reveal a plasmacytoma within left parietal bone marrow, which destroyed the inner and outer skull tables, in an elderly woman. Extraosseous extension is present. (Source: Introduction. In: Meyers S, ed. Differential Diagnosis in Neuroimaging: Brain and Meninges. 1st ed. Thieme; 2016).

## 8.4.5 Treatment Options

- Acute pain control with medications and pain management
- If tumor is metastatic:
  - Tumor resection surgery (if located in a single area of the brain) followed by radiation therapy
  - Radiation therapy (i.e., WBRT)
  - Immunotherapy (i.e., Yervoy, Opdivo, Keytruda)
  - Intracranial chemotherapy or catheter-mediated chemotherapy (for leptomeningeal metastases); radiation therapy may also be used
  - Targeted therapy
    - Tagrisso for NSCLC with genetic alteration to EGFR gene

- ○ Alecensa for NSCLC with genetic alteration to ALK gene
- ○ Tykerb for HER2-positive breast cancer
- ○ Tafinlar and/or Mekinist and Zelboraf for melanoma
- If tumor is deemed low grade and can be fully removed in one step (tumor is focused in one area):
  - – Tumor resection surgery
    - ○ Radiation therapy may be required if tumor cannot be fully removed
    - ○ Transnasal endoscopic surgery if small and easily reachable (typically for olfactory groove meningioma)
    - ○ Craniotomy or minicraniotomy approaches (removing part of the skull to resect tumor)
    - ○ Pterional approach (shortest route to suprasellar cisterns)
    - ○ Transsphenoidal approach (most common for pituitary gland tumors)
    - ○ Endoscopic approach (an endoscope is a tube with an inbuilt microscope, light, and camera that a surgeon can insert instruments through for tumor resection)
    - ○ Embolization performed prior to surgery if meningioma is large and has rich vascular supply
- If tumor is deemed high grade and cannot be fully removed by surgery:
  - – Tumor resection surgery if deemed suitable candidate for surgery; may be followed by radiation treatment and chemotherapy (may be supplemented by target therapy) after resection if considered necessary by the radiation oncologist
    - ○ Oncologist will need to determine overall prognosis, Karnofsky performance score, and extent of visceral disease
    - ○ If poor surgical candidate with poor life expectancy, medical management recommended
  - – Radiation therapy
    - ○ Conventional radiation therapy
    - ○ 3D-CRT
    - ○ IMRT
    - ○ Proton therapy
    - ○ Radiosurgery/CyberKnife treatment (primary treatment for metastases)
- If pituitary gland is not making enough hormone:
  - – Hormone replacement therapy (HRT)
    - ○ Replacement of: thyroid, adrenal, growth, testosterone (men), and/or estrogen (women)
- If pituitary gland is making too much hormone:
  - – Drug therapy
    - ○ Prolactin oversecretion: bromocriptine (Parlodel) and cabergoline (Dostinex)

- Growth hormone oversecretion: octreotide (Sandostatin) or pegvisomant (Somavert)
- Thyroid-stimulating hormone oversecretion: ocreotide (Sandostatin)

## 8.4.6 Indications for Surgical Intervention

- No improvement after nonoperative therapy (physical therapy, pain management, radiation treatment, and chemotherapy)
- Large tumor of over 3 cm causing significant mass effect or obstructive hydrocephalus
- Patient does not possess more than four brain lesions from multiple metastases
- Tumor surgically accessible
- Tumor recurrence following other treatments
- Residual tumor(s) present after surgery
- Presence of pituitary adenoma, craniopharyngioma, Rathke's cleft cyst, meningioma, or chordoma causing mass effect or vision disturbance

## 8.4.7 Surgical Procedure for Transsphenoidal Endoscopic Pituitary

1. Informed consent signed, preoperative labs normal, patient ceases intaking of NSAIDs (Naprosyn, Advil, Nuprin, Motrin, Aleve) and blood thinners (Coumadin, Plavix, Aspirin) 1 week prior to treatment
2. Prep patient's nose with antibiotic and antiseptic solutions
3. Appropriate intubation and sedation and lines (if necessary) as per the anesthetist
4. Place image-guidance system on patient's head
5. Neuromonitoring not needed
6. Time out is performed with agreement from everyone in the room for correct patient and correct surgery with consent signed
7. Insert endoscope into a nostril and progress it to the back of nasal cavity
8. Remove small portion of nasal septum dividing left and right nostril
9. Open sphenoid sinus using bone-biting instruments
10. Remove the thin bone of the sella, exposing the dura
11. Open the dura, exposing the tumor and pituitary gland
12. Remove the tumor in pieces through a small hole in the sella, using long grasping instruments
    a. Core out the center of tumor so that the margins fall inward and become surgically accessible
    b. After visible tumor is resected, move endoscope into sella to search for hidden tumor portions (i.e., in cavernous sinus)
    c. If a tumor cannot be safely removed, radiation therapy may be used later

13. Close the sella opening:
    a. Perform a 2 cm skin incision in the abdomen to obtain a fat graft, if deemed appropriate and necessary. Fill the space the tumor previously occupied with this graft. Suture abdominal incision
    b. Replace hole in sella floor with bone graft from septum (or from synthetic graft material). Apply biologic glue over graft in sphenoid sinus
14. Close all skin incisions with sutures or surgical staples
15. Apply sterile bandage or dressing over incisions

## 8.4.8 Pitfalls

- CSF rhinorrhea
- Meningitis
- Surgically induced pituitary damage
- Diabetes insipidus
- Major bleeding
- Vision abnormalities

## 8.4.9 Prognosis

- Hospitalization rates depend on the type of procedure performed, preoperative examination status, and patient's age/comorbidities
- Aftercare at home after discharge
- Pain management
- Headache, nausea, or vomiting, if present following the procedure, will warrant relevant medications

# 8.5 Superficial Tumor Resection (Arising from Skull)

## 8.5.1 Symptoms and Signs (Broad)

- Incidental with symptoms (depending on size and location)
- Headaches progressively increasing in frequency and severity
- Nausea and/or vomiting
- Blurred vision, double vision, or loss of peripheral vision
- Difficulty maintaining balance
- Reduction in sensation or motor control of certain extremities
- Difficulty producing speech
- Changes in behavior/reduction in awareness
- Seizures (especially associated with superficial tumors)
- Reduction in hearing capabilities
- Skull erosion

## 8.5.2 Surgical Pathology

- Cranial benign/malignant tumor

## 8.5.3 Diagnostic Modalities

- Physical examination
- Neurological examination
- Cerebral angiography DTI
- SPECT of brain
- MRI of brain (see ▶ Fig. 8.10 and ▶ Fig. 8.11)
- PET scan of brain
- Optical in vivo imaging (involving bioluminescence and fluorescence)
- Biopsy of tissue

## 8.5.4 Differential Diagnosis

- Metastatic tumor
  - Breast, colon, lung, melanoma, renal cell
- Primary tumor (may become metastatic)
  - Glioma
    ○ Astrocytoma (astrocytomas, anaplastic astrocytomas, glioblastomas)
    ○ Oligodendroglial
    ○ Mixed glioma (both astrocytic and oligodenrocytic)
  - Meningioma
    ○ Grade I (slow growth, distinct borders)

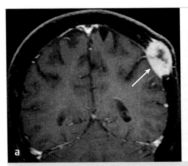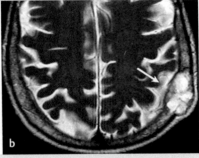

**Fig. 8.10 (a, b)** MRI scans reveal metastatic breast carcinoma with numerous skull marrow lesions in an elderly woman. Extraosseous extension is present. (Source: Diseases affecting the temporal bone. In: Tsementzis S, ed. Differential Diagnosis in Neurology and Neurosurgery: A Clinician's Pocket Guide. 2nd ed. Thieme; 2019).

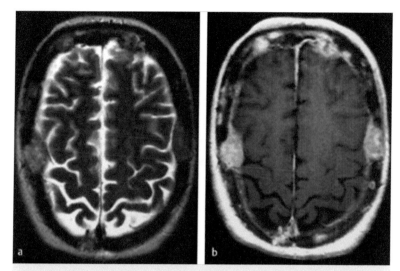

**Fig. 8.11** (a, b) MRI scans reveal metastatic breast carcinoma with numerous skull marrow lesions in an elderly woman. Extraosseous extension is present. (Source: Zenga J, Sharon J, Santiago P, et al. Lower trapezius flap for reconstruction of posterior scalp and neck defects after complex occipital-cervical surgeries. J Neurol Surg B Skull Base 2015;76(5):397–408).

- Grade II (atypical)
- Grade III (malignant/cancerous)
- Dermoid tumor

## 8.5.5 Treatment Options

- Acute pain control with medications and pain management
- If tumor is metastatic:
  - Tumor resection surgery (if located in a single area of the brain) followed by radiation therapy
  - Radiation therapy (i.e., WBRT)
  - Immunotherapy (i.e., Yervoy, Opdivo, Keytruda)
  - Intracranial chemotherapy or catheter-mediated chemotherapy (for leptomeningeal metastases); radiation therapy may also be used
  - Targeted therapy
    - Tagrisso for NSCLC with genetic alteration to EGFR gene
    - Alecensa for NSCLC with genetic alteration to ALK gene

- o Tykerb for HER2-positive breast cancer
- o Tafinlar and/or Mekinist and Zelboraf for melanoma
- If tumor is deemed low grade and can be fully removed in one step (tumor is focused in one area):
  - – Tumor resection surgery
    - o Radiation therapy may be required if tumor cannot be fully removed
    - o Transnasal endoscopic surgery if small and easily reachable (typically for olfactory groove meningioma)
    - o Craniotomy or minicraniotomy approaches (removing part of the skull to resect tumor)
    - o Pterional approach (shortest route to suprasellar cisterns)
    - o Embolization performed prior to surgery if meningioma is large and has rich vascular supply
- If tumor is deemed high grade and cannot be fully removed by surgery:
  - – Tumor resection surgery if deemed suitable candidate for surgery; may be followed by radiation treatment and chemotherapy (may be supplemented by target therapy) after resection if considered necessary by the radiation oncologist
    - o Oncologist will need to determine overall prognosis, Karnofsky performance score, and extent of visceral disease
    - o If poor surgical candidate with poor life expectancy, medical management recommended
  - – Radiation therapy
    - o Conventional radiation therapy
    - o 3D-CRT
    - o IMRT
    - o Proton therapy
    - o Radiosurgery/CyberKnife treatment (primary treatment for metastases)

## 8.5.6 Indications for Surgical Intervention

- No improvement after nonoperative therapy (physical therapy, pain management, radiation treatment, and chemotherapy)
- Metastasis in single brain location
- Large tumor(s) of over 3 cm causing significant mass effect or obstructive hydrocephalus
- Patient does not possess more than four brain lesions from multiple metastases
- Tumor(s) surgically accessible
- Tumor recurrence following other treatments
- Residual tumor(s) present after surgery

## 8.5.7 Surgical Procedure for Craniotomy

1. Informed consent signed, preoperative labs normal, patient ceases intaking of NSAIDs (Naprosyn, Advil, Nuprin, Motrin, Aleve) and blood thinners (Coumadin, Plavix, Aspirin) 1 week prior to treatment
2. Appropriate intubation and sedation and lines (if necessary) as per the anesthetist
3. Patient's head is shaved and skin overlaying surgical site is cleansed with antiseptic solution
4. Place patient in a position appropriate for reaching the tumor location on operating table, with Mayfield Pin fixation, and all pressure points padded
5. Neuromonitoring not needed
6. Time out is performed with agreement from everyone in the room for correct patient and correct surgery with consent signed
7. Incise skin in location appropriate for reaching the location of tumor
8. Pull the scalp up and clip it to control bleeding, allowing access to brain
9. Make burr holes in the skull using a medical drill and carefully cut the bone using a saw, if necessary
10. Remove the bone flap, saving it for future steps
11. Extracerebral tumors are commonly firmly attached to the dura
12. Separate the dura mater from the bone and cut it, exposing the brain, if deemed appropriate and necessary
13. Remove the tumor for gross total resection
14. Ensure that all surgically accessible tumor components have been resected
    a. If tumor components remain, radiotherapy may be performed later
15. Suture the appropriate layers of tissue
16. Reattach the bone flap using plates, sutures, or wires
    a. If a tumor or infection is present in the bone, do not reattach it
    b. If decompression is required, do not reattach the bone flap
17. Close skin incision with sutures or surgical staples
18. Apply sterile bandage or dressing over incision

## 8.5.8 Pitfalls

- Recurrence of tumor(s) after surgery
- Neurologic deficits
- Acute respiratory failure
- Brain swelling
- Paralysis, memory deficits, difficulty producing speech, diminished balance, and/or coma (rare)

### 8.5.9 Prognosis

- Patient will be taken to a recovery room and ultimately to the ICU. Hospitalization rates depend on the type of procedure performed, preoperative examination status, and patient's age/comorbidities
- Patient will have to enroll in rehabilitation unit for several days after hospital stay, if necessary
- Patient will have SCDs placed on legs while in bed to reduce chance of blood clot formation
- Headache, nausea, or vomiting, if present following the procedure, will warrant relevant medications

## 8.6 Epidural Tumor Resection

### 8.6.1 Symptoms and Signs (Broad)

- Incidental with symptoms (depending on size and location)
- Headaches progressively increasing in frequency and severity
- Nausea and/or vomiting
- Blurred vision, double vision, or loss of peripheral vision
- Difficulty maintaining balance
- Reduction in sensation or motor control of certain extremities
- Difficulty producing speech
- Changes in behavior/reduction in awareness
- Seizures (especially associated with superficial tumors)
- Reduction in hearing capabilities
- Skull erosion
- Hydrocephalus

### 8.6.2 Surgical Pathology

- Cranial benign/malignant tumor

### 8.6.3 Diagnostic Modalities

- Physical examination
- Neurological examination
- Cerebral angiography DTI
- SPECT of brain
- MRI of brain (see ▶ Fig. 8.12)
- PET scan of brain
- Optical in vivo imaging (involving bioluminescence and fluorescence)
- Biopsy of tissue

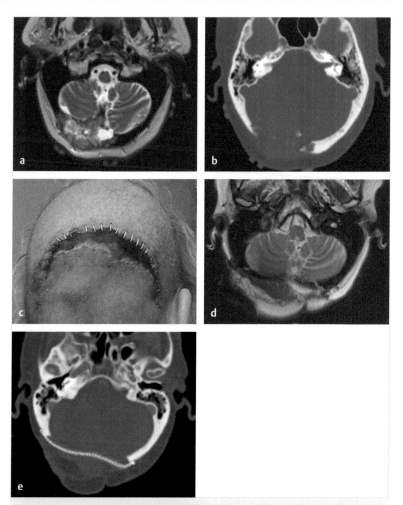

**Fig. 8.12** Preoperative MRI scans revealed large lesion, sella erosion, and calcifications in a 4-year-old girl (**a–c**). An epidural tumor was pushing dura toward the foramen of Monro. Postoperative images (3 weeks) demonstrate pterional removal (**d, e**) and neurological recovery was achieved. (Source: Cases. In: Yasargil M, ed. Microneurosurgery, Vol. IV A. CNS Tumors: Surgical Anatomy, Neuropathology, Neuroradiology, Neurophysiology, Clinical Considerations, Operability, Treatment Options. 1st ed. Thieme; 1994).

## 8.6.4 Differential Diagnosis

- Metastatic tumor
  - Breast, colon, lung, melanoma, renal cell
- Primary tumor
  - Glioma
    - Astrocytoma (astrocytomas, anaplastic astrocytomas, glioblastomas)
    - Oligodendroglial
    - Mixed glioma (both astrocytic and oligodenrocytic)
  - Meningioma
    - Grade I (slow growth, distinct borders)
    - Grade II (atypical)
    - Grade III (malignant/cancerous)
  - Schwannoma
  - Craniopharyngioma
  - Pituitary
  - Primary lymphoma
  - Choroid plexus papilloma/carcinoma
  - Dermoid tumor
  - Hemangioblastoma
  - Posterior fossa tumor
    - Medulloblastoma
    - Pineoblastoma
    - Ependymoma
    - PNET
    - Astrocytoma of cerebellum and brainstem

## 8.6.5 Treatment Options

- Acute pain control with medications and pain management
- If tumor is metastatic:
  - Tumor resection surgery (if located in a single area of the brain) followed by radiation therapy if necessary
  - Radiation therapy (i.e., WBRT) if multiple lesions
  - Immunotherapy (i.e., Yervoy, Opdivo, Keytruda)
  - Intracranial chemotherapy or catheter-mediated chemotherapy (for leptomeningeal metastases); radiation therapy may also be used
  - Targeted therapy
    - Tagrisso for NSCLC with genetic alteration to EGFR gene
    - Alecensa for NSCLC with genetic alteration to ALK gene

- o Tykerb for HER2-positive breast cancer
- o Tafinlar and/or Mekinist and Zelboraf for melanoma
- If tumor is deemed low grade and can be fully removed in one step (tumor is focused in one area):
  - – Tumor resection surgery
    - o Radiation therapy may be required if tumor cannot be fully removed
    - o Transnasal endoscopic surgery if small and easily reachable (typically for olfactory groove meningioma and pituitary tumors)
    - o Craniotomy or minicraniotomy approaches (removing part of the skull to resect tumor) (see ▶ Fig. 8.13)
    - o Pterional approach (shortest route to suprasellar cisterns)
    - o Embolization performed prior to surgery if meningioma is large and has rich vascular supply
- If tumor is deemed high grade and cannot be fully removed by surgery:
  - – Tumor resection surgery if deemed suitable candidate for surgery; may be followed by radiation treatment and chemotherapy (may be supplemented by target therapy) after resection if considered necessary by the radiation oncologist
    - o Oncologist will need to determine overall prognosis, Karnofsky performance score, and extent of visceral disease
    - o If poor surgical candidate with poor life expectancy, medical management recommended
  - – Radiation therapy
    - o Conventional radiation therapy
    - o 3D-CRT
    - o IMRT
    - o Proton therapy
    - o Radiosurgery/CyberKnife treatment (primary treatment for metastases)

## 8.6.6 Indications for Surgical Intervention

- No improvement after nonoperative therapy (physical therapy, pain management, radiation treatment, and chemotherapy)
- Large tumor(s) of over 3 cm causing significant mass effect or obstructive hydrocephalus
- Patient does not possess more than four brain lesions from multiple metastases
- Tumor(s) surgically accessible
- Tumor recurrence following other treatments
- Residual tumor(s) present after surgery

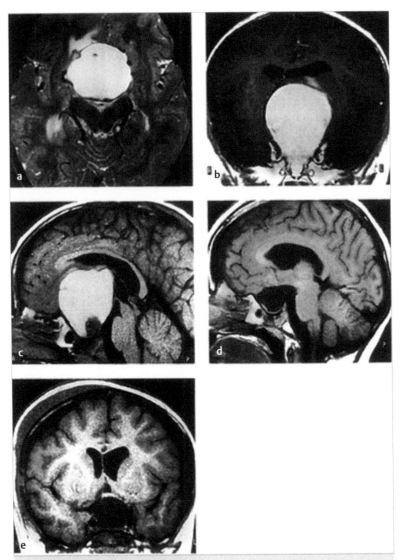

**Fig. 8.13** Preoperative MRI scans revealed large lesion, sella erosion, and calcifications in a 4-year-old girl (**a–c**). An epidural tumor was pushing dura toward the foramen of Monro. Postoperative images (3 weeks) demonstrate pterional removal (**d, e**) and neurological recovery was achieved.

## 8.6.7 Surgical Procedure for Retrosigmoid Craniotomy (Meningiomas or Vestibular Schwannomas)

1. Informed consent signed, preoperative labs normal, patient ceases intaking of NSAIDs (Naprosyn, Advil, Nuprin, Motrin, Aleve) and blood thinners (Coumadin, Plavix, Aspirin) 1 week prior to treatment
2. Appropriate intubation and sedation and lines (if necessary) as per the anesthetist
3. Place patient in lateral park bench position with rigid head fixation using Mayfield Pin skull clamp, all pressure points padded, and axillary roll placed
4. Rotate patient's head 10–15 degrees toward contralateral side, neck minimally flexed
5. Cleanse patient's skin overlaying surgical site with antiseptic solution
6. Neuromonitoring may be required to monitor nerves (if necessary and indicated)
7. Time out is performed with agreement from everyone in the room for correct patient and correct surgery with consent signed
8. Create curvilinear incision behind the ear, to provide access to cerebellum and brainstem
   a. Incision made about 2.5 fingerbreadths behind postauricular sulcus
9. Reach bone using scalpel and monopolar cautery, placing self-retaining retractors
10. Locate the asterion and perform a 4 cm craniotomy posterior and inferior to sigmoid and transverse sinus, respectively
11. Drill a circumferential trough using a M8 bit
12. Turn and elevate the bone flap
    a. If appropriate extradural exposure of transverse and sigmoid sinuses is not reached, further drilling may be necessary
13. Wax bone edges to minimize risk of CSF leakage postoperatively
14. Plug any emissary veins with bone wax or bipolar coagulation
15. Obtain hemostasis and open the dura with a curvilinear incision, 3–5 mm away from margin of transverse-sigmoid sinus
    a. Cover this dural leaf with moist towel and tack it using 4-0 Nurolon
16. Place retractor and allow CSF to egress from foramen magnum
17. Gently retract cerebellum medially and divide any imposing arachnoid bands
18. Bipolar coagulate and resect a leaf of dura at future site of drilling, over posterior petrous temporal bone
19. Remove all cottonoids and pledgets from the field and place Gelfoam in the cistern

20. Start resecting tumor (meningioma or schwannoma)
21. For remaining tumor, drill the bone away until the lateral internal auditory canal is identified:
    a. Use a 3 mm cutting burr, progressing to a two diamond drill when approaching the internal auditory canal
    b. Develop superior and inferior troughs until the internal auditory canal is exposed by about 270 degrees
    c. "Blue line" the posterior canal and vestibule for lateral extending tumors
22. Test the posterior capsule of tumor with flush-tip Prass probe, ensuring facial nerve is following ventral course
23. Open internal auditory canal dura and reflect the dural leaflets superiorly and inferiorly
24. Internally debulk the tumor using bipolar electrocautery and tumor forceps, and dissect the capsule free from facial and cochlear nerves
    a. Be very careful when employing bipolar coagulation and neurovascular traction
    b. Use a 30-degree rigid endoscope to confirm complete tumor resection involving the lateral internal auditory canal
    c. Occlude any perimeatal air cells with bone wax
    d. Occlude fundus with fascia/muscle plug
    e. A small sheen of capsule is left and microdissected off the facial nerve
25. Irrigate wound with saline and remove retractors
26. Close dura in watertight fashion using 4–0 Nurolon suture
27. Place Gelfoam on top of dura
28. Replace bone flap with KLS screws and plates
29. Use methylmethacrylate to close the remainder of cranial opening
30. Irrigate wound with Bacitracin irrigation and close in layers with 2–0 Vicryls in multiple layers in muscle, 3–0 Vicryls in galea and dermis, and a running, locked 3–0 nylon in skin

## 8.6.8 Pitfalls

- Recurrence of tumor(s) after surgery
- Neurologic deficits
- Hearing loss
- Epidural hematoma
- Brain swelling
- Paralysis, memory deficits, difficulty producing speech, diminished balance, and/or coma (rare)
- CSF leakage

## 8.6.9 Prognosis

- Patient will be taken to a recovery room and ultimately to the ICU. Hospitalization rates depend on the type of procedure performed, preoperative examination status, and patient's age/comorbidities
- Patient will have to enroll in rehabilitation unit for several days after hospital stay, if necessary
- Patient will have SCDs placed on legs while in bed to reduce chance of blood clot formation
- Headache, nausea, or vomiting, if present following the procedure, will warrant relevant medications

# Bibliography

Al-Shatoury H, Galhom A, Engelhard H. Posterior Fossa Tumors Treatment & Management. Medscape. 2018. (https://emedicine.medscape.com/article/249495-treatment)

Chung HJ, Park JS, Park JH, Jeun SS. Remote postoperative epidural hematoma after brain tumor surgery. Brain Tumor Res Treat 2015;3(2):132–137

Convexity Meningioma. Mount Sinai. (https://www.mountsinai.org/care/neurosurgery/services/meningiomas/types/convexity)

Olfactory Groove Meningioma. Mount Sinai. (https://www.mountsinai.org/care/neurosurgery/services/meningiomas/types/olfactory-groove)

Craniotomy. Johns Hopkins Medicine. (https://www.hopkinsmedicine.org/healthlibrary/test_procedures/neurological/craniotomy_92,p08767)

Endoscopic Pituitary Surgery. Johns Hopkins Medicine. (https://www.hopkinsmedicine.org/healthlibrary/test_procedures/neurological/endoscopic_pituitary_surgery_135,42)

Farooq G, Rehman L, Bokhari I, Rizvi SRH. Modern microsurgical resection of olfactory groove meningiomas by classical bicoronal subfrontal approach without orbital osteotomies. Asian J Neurosurg 2018;13(2):258–263

Forbes J, Carlson M, Godil S, Bennett M, Wanna G, Weaver K. Retrosigmoid craniotomy for resection of acoustic neuroma with hearing preservation: a video publication. Neurosurg Focus (Suppl) 2014;36:Video 8

Hatiboglu MA, Wildrick DM, Sawaya R. The role of surgical resection in patients with brain metastases. Ecancermedicalscience 2013;7:308

Marburger T, Prayson R. Angiocentric glioma: a clinicopathologic review of 5 tumors with identification of associated cortical dysplasia. Arch Pathol Lab Med 2011;135(8):1037–1041

Mishra RC, Mishra S. Olfactory groove meningiomas: the surgical approaches and factors influencing prognosis. Neurol India 2018;66(4):964–966

Pituitary Gland Tumor: Symptoms and Signs. Cancer.Net. 2017. (https://www.cancer.net/cancer-types/pituitary-gland-tumor/symptoms-and-signs)

Pituitary Gland Tumor: Treatment Options. Cancer.Net. 2017. (https://www.cancer.net/cancer-types/pituitary-gland-tumor/treatment-options)

Taratuto AL, Monges J, Lylyk P, Leiguarda R. Superficial cerebral astrocytoma attached to dura. Report of six cases in infants. Cancer 1984;54(11):2505–2512

Zimmer L, DiNapoli V. Endoscopic pituitary surgery (transsphenoidal). Mayfield Brain & Spine. 2018. (https://mayfieldclinic.com/pe-endopitsurg.htm)

# 9 Cerebral Vascular Lesions

*Ryan F. Amidon, Christ Ordookhanian, and Paul E. Kaloostian*

## 9.1 Cerebral Aneurysms/Cerebral AVM Resection/Cerebral Cavernous Angioma Resection

### 9.1.1 Symptoms and Signs

- Headaches progressively increasing in frequency and severity
- Nausea and/or vomiting
- Lack of appetite
- Neck pain/stiffness
- Blurred vision, double vision, or loss of peripheral vision
- Seizures
- Loss of memory or confusion
- Reduction in hearing capabilities
- Fever
- Difficulty maintaining balance and properly performing movements
- Unilateral paralysis
- Weakness/Numbness in arm/leg
- Difficulty speaking
- Cognitive deficiency

### 9.1.2 Surgical Pathology

- Cranial benign/malignant vascular lesion

### 9.1.3 Diagnostic Modalities

- Physical examination
- Neurological examination
- Cerebral angiography(see ▶ Fig. 9.1)
- MRI of brain (if positive, angiogram performed)
- CT scan of brain (if positive, angiogram performed)

### 9.1.4 Differential Diagnosis

- Arteriovenous malformation (AVM)
- Cavernoma (cavernous angioma) (see ▶ Fig. 9.2)

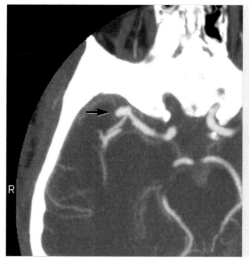

**Fig. 9.1** Image of ruptured cerebral aneurysm that resulted in subarachnoid hemorrhage. (Source: Intracerebral aneurysms. In: Ryan D, ed. Handbook of Neuroscience Nursing: Care of the Adult Neurosurgical Patient. 1st ed. Thieme; 2019).

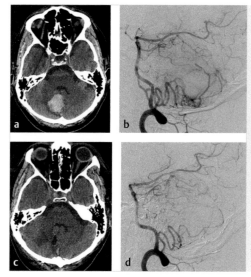

**Fig. 9.2** CT scan (**a**) and cerebral angiography (**b**) revealed right cerebellar hemorrhage and AVM. The patient received AVM excision and hematoma evacuation and follow-up images demonstrate total AVM resection (**c**, **d**). (Source: Indications and contraindications for surgery. In: Macdonald R, ed. Neurosurgical Operative Atlas: Vascular Neurosurgery. 3rd ed. Thieme; 2018).

- Mixed malformation
- Dural arteriovenous fistula (DAVF)
- Telangiectasis
  - Capillary telangiectasia (CTS)

- Venous malformation
  - Developmental venous anomaly (DVA)
- Vein of Galen malformation
- Cerebral aneurysm (see ▶ Fig. 9.3)
- Moyamoya disease

## 9.1.5 Treatment Options

- Conservative observation
- Radiation therapy
  - Conventional radiation therapy
  - Three-dimensional conformal radiation therapy (3D-CRT)
  - Intensity modulated radiation therapy (IMRT)
  - Proton therapy
  - Radiosurgery/CyberKnife treatment
- Surgery
  - Microsurgical resection
  - Preferred option if bleeding or seizures result from lesion

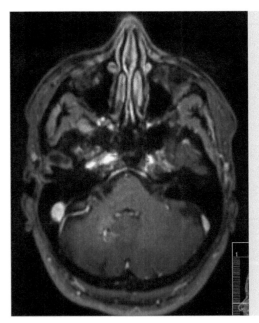

**Fig. 9.3** MRI scan reveals cavernous angioma in cerebellar hemisphere. (Source: Cranial. In: Shaya M, Gragnaniello C, Nader R, eds. Neurosurgery Rounds: Questions and Answers. 2nd ed. Thieme; 2017).

- Endovascular embolization using the following embolic agents (initial procedure to facilitate surgery):
  - Coils: Close down vessel supplying AVM (cannot independently treat AVM nidus)
  - Onyx: Solidifies, forming a cast, in vessel supplying AVM (best penetration of AVM nidus)
  - NBCA: Solidifies as a glue in vessel supplying AVM (greater risks and worse outcomes than with Onyx)
  - PVA: Used prior to craniotomy or surgical resection of AVM (cannot independently treat AVM pathology)
- Combination techniques
  - Embolization followed by stereotactic radiosurgery
- Venous angiomas should not be treated unless certainly contributing to intractable seizures and bleeding

## 9.1.6 Indications for Surgical Intervention

- No improvement after nonoperative therapy (physical therapy, pain management, radiation treatment, and chemotherapy)
- Palliative treatment when symptomatic vascular lesion not entirely treatable by other approaches
- Vascular lesion surgically accessible, sufficiently small, and near surface of brain
- Presence of associated lesions (aneurysms/pseudoaneurysms on feeding pedicle or nidus, venous thrombosis, venous outflow restriction, venous pouches, dilatations)

## 9.1.7 Surgical Procedure for Microsurgical Resection (Vascular Lesions)

1. Informed consent signed, preoperative labs normal, patient ceases intake of NSAIDs (Naprosyn, Advil, Nuprin, Motrin, Aleve) and blood thinners (Coumadin, Plavix, Aspirin) 1 week prior to treatment
2. Appropriate intubation and sedation and lines (if necessary) as per the anesthetist
3. Place patient in supine position with Mayfield pins, all pressure points padded, and head turned to relevant side of vascular lesion
4. Cleanse patient's skin overlaying surgical site with antiseptic solution
5. Neuromonitoring may be present to monitor nerves
6. Time out is performed with agreement from everyone in the room for correct patient and correct surgery with consent signed

7. Perform arched incision on scalp along AVM/vascular lesion (cavernoma, etc.), folding soft tissue back
8. Drill small holes in the skull and create a skull flap (craniotomy)
9. Open the dura, allowing direct access to vascular lesion
10. IF AVM, separate AVM and clamp the blood vessels on both sides of the malformation, cutting off blood circulation to the abnormal vessels, starting with supplying arteries then nidus and finally the draining veins
11. If cavernoma, remove the cavernoma en bloc by separating mass from surrounding parenchyma of brain
12. If aneurysm, carefully isolate the aneurysm neck with proximal and distal arterial control prior to placing appropriate clips across neck (given preoperative preparation demonstrates this aneurysm to be favorable for clipping with large neck rather than endovascular treatment needing smaller neck of aneurysm)
13. Carefully free and surgically remove AVM/vascular lesion
14. A drain may be placed at the surgical site, preventing fluid build-up
15. Ensure that the AVM/vascular lesion is entirely resected
16. Close dura in watertight fashion
17. Return or replace skull flap, using screws and plates if necessary
18. Seal back the skin flap with surgical staples or sutures

## 9.1.8 Embolization Procedure (Onyx)

1. Shake Onyx vial on mixer for 20 minutes. Onyx-18 is common, Onyx-34 is suitable for very high-flow AVMs, and Onyx-500 is incorporated in aneurysm embolization treatments
2. Wedge microcatheter tip into arterial branch supplying the AVM, preferably very close to the AVM nidus
3. Perform angiography through the microcatheter to confirm that the arterial branch exclusively supplies the AVM
4. Prime the DMSO-compatible microcatheter (marathon, echelon, rebar, ultraflow) with 0.3 to 0.8 mL DMSO so that Onyx does not solidify in the microcatheter
5. Slowly inject Onyx solution, allowing no more than 1 cm of reflux. If reflux occurs, continue after 1 to 2 minute waiting period
6. Halt injection when Onyx no longer flows into the nidus, but refluxes instead

## 9.1.9 Pitfalls

- Neurocognitive deficits
- Continued bleeding after surgery

- Local brain swelling
- Failure to remove entire vascular lesion source
- Future recurrence of vascular lesion
- Damage to cranial nerve(s)
- Risk of surgery related to the size of vascular lesion, deep venous drainage, lenticulostriate arterial supply, and diffuse nidus

## 9.1.10 Prognosis

- Patient will be taken to a recovery room and ultimately to the ICU for several days. Hospitalization rates depend on the type of procedure performed, preoperative examination status, and patient's age/comorbidities
- Patient will have to enroll in rehabilitation unit for several days after hospital stay, if necessary
- Headache, nausea, or vomiting, if present following the procedure, will warrant relevant medications

# 9.2 Endovascular Treatment of Cerebral Aneurysms/AVM

## 9.2.1 Symptoms and Signs

- Headaches progressively increasing in frequency and severity
- Nausea and/or vomiting
- Lack of appetite
- Neck pain/stiffness
- Blurred vision, double vision, or loss of peripheral vision
- Seizures
- Loss of memory or confusion
- Reduction in hearing capabilities
- Fever
- Difficulty maintaining balance and properly performing movements
- Unilateral paralysis
- Weakness/numbness in arm/leg
- Difficulty speaking
- Cognitive deficiency
- Facial pain

## 9.2.2 Surgical Pathology

- Cranial benign/malignant vascular lesion

## 9.2.3 Diagnostic Modalities

- Physical examination
- Neurological examination
- Cerebral angiography (see ▶ Fig. 9.4)
- MRI of brain (if positive, angiogram performed)
- CT scan of brain (if positive, angiogram performed)

## 9.2.4 Differential Diagnosis AVM

- Cavernoma (cavernous angioma)
- Mixed malformation
- DAVF
- Telangiectasis CTS
- Venous malformation DVA
- Vein of Galen malformation
- Moyamoya disease

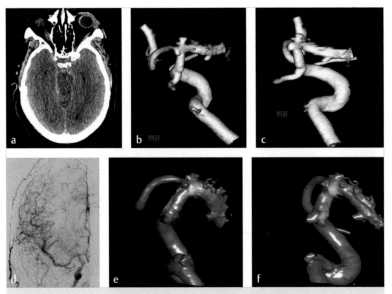

Fig. 9.4 CT scan revealed a subarachnoid hemorrhage in a middle-aged woman suffering from severe headache (a). Catheter angiography revealed two irregular aneurysms at the internal carotid artery (ICA) and middle cerebral artery (MCA) (b–d). She received endovascular treatment and aneurysm coverage was confirmed with postplacement angiography (e, f).

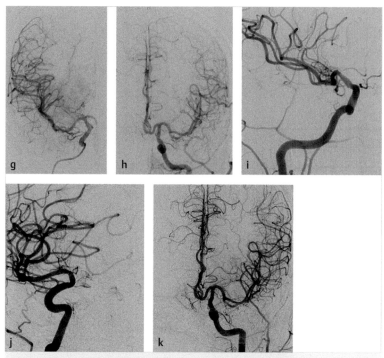

**Fig. 9.4** (*Continued*) Postplacement angiography also demonstrated heightened cross-filling of the anterior cerebral artery (ACA) (**g, h**). Follow-up angiography (1 year) confirmed total occlusion of aneurysm (**i, j**). ACA filling from left carotid injection was also confirmed (**k**). (Source: Ruptured aneurysms. In: Park M, Taussky P, Albuquerque F, et al, eds. Flow Diversion of Cerebral Aneurysms. 1st ed. Thieme; 2017).

## 9.2.5 Treatment Options

- Conservative observation
- Radiation therapy
  - Conventional radiation therapy
  - 3D-CRT
  - IMRT
  - Proton therapy
  - Radiosurgery/CyberKnife treatment
- Surgery
  - Microsurgical resection
  - Preferred option if bleeding or seizures result from lesion

- Endovascular embolization using the following embolic agents (initial procedure to facilitate surgery):
  - Coils: Close down vessel supplying AVM (not the best for AVM nidus)
  - Onyx: Solidifies, forming a cast, in vessel supplying AVM (best penetration of AVM nidus)
  - NBCA: Solidifies as a glue in vessel supplying AVM (greater risks and worse outcomes than with Onyx)
  - PVA: Used prior to craniotomy or surgical resection of AVM (cannot independently treat AVM pathology)
- Combination techniques
  - Surgery/Embolization followed by stereotactic radiosurgery
- Venous angiomas should not be treated unless certainly contributing to intractable seizures and bleeding

## 9.2.6 Indications for Surgical Intervention

- No improvement after nonoperative therapy (physical therapy, pain management, radiation treatment)
- Palliative treatment when symptomatic vascular lesion not entirely treatable by other approaches
- Vascular lesion surgically accessible, sufficiently small, and near surface of brain
- Presence of associated lesions (aneurysms/pseudoaneurysms on feeding pedicle or nidus, venous thrombosis, venous outflow restriction, venous pouches, dilatations)

## 9.2.7 Surgical Procedure for Endovascular Embolization (Coiling)

1. Informed consent signed, preoperative labs normal, patient ceases intake of NSAIDs (Naprosyn, Advil, Nuprin, Motrin, Aleve) and blood thinners (Coumadin, Plavix, Aspirin) 1 week prior to treatment
2. Appropriate intubation and sedation and lines (if necessary) as per the anesthetist
3. Place patient in supine position in interventional radiology (IR) suite, all pressure points padded, and head neutral
4. Cleanse patient's skin overlaying femoral groin site with antiseptic solution
5. Neuromonitoring not needed
6. Catheter may be placed in patient's bladder to drain urine
7. Time out is performed with agreement from everyone in the room for correct patient and correct surgery with consent signed

8. Insert catheter through groin toward vascular lesion source:
   a. Perform incision in skin, exposing artery in groin
   b. Insert catheter into artery using guide wire and fluoroscopic guidance
   c. Once catheter reaches affected artery, inject contrast dye to visualize via X-ray fluoroscopy
   d. Measure aneurysm, recording its properties (i.e., shape)
   e. Insert a smaller catheter into the original catheter toward aneurysm
   f. Once aneurysm is reached, move coil or glue into aneurysm
   g. Once the coil is entirely within aneurysm, release it from catheter
      i. Place as many coils as necessary to seal off aneurysm
      ii. Take X-ray images to ensure the aneurysm is sealed off
      iii. Coil(s) left in place
   h. Remove catheter
9. Achieve proper hemostasis and apply dressing

## 9.2.8 Pitfalls

- Allergies to dye used for X-ray visualization or iodine
- Neurocognitive deficits
- Continued bleeding after surgery, particularly in pregnant patients and those taking anticoagulants
- Aneurysm
- Stroke
- Unilateral paralysis
- Blood clot or hematoma (significant likelihood in groin, where catheter is inserted)
- Aphasia
- Infection
- Failure to remove entire vascular lesion source
- Future recurrence of vascular lesion
- Damage to cranial nerve(s)
- Risk of surgery related to the size of vascular lesion, deep venous drainage, lenticulostriate arterial supply, and diffuse nidus

## 9.2.9 Prognosis

- Patient will be taken to a recovery room and ultimately to the ICU for several days. Hospitalization rates depend on the type of procedure performed, preoperative examination status, and patient's age/comorbidities
- Remain flat in bed for 12 to 24 hours after procedure

- Patient will have to enroll in rehabilitation unit for several days after hospital stay, if necessary
- Headache, nausea, or vomiting, if present following the procedure, will warrant relevant medications

# Bibliography

AVM Resection. The American Center for Spine & Neurosurgery. 2019. (http://www.acsneuro.com/surgeries/brain_detail/avm_resection)

Davidson AS, Morgan MK. How safe is arteriovenous malformation surgery? A prospective, observational study of surgery as first-line treatment for brain arteriovenous malformations. Neurosurgery 2010;66(3):498–504, discussion 504–505

Endovascular Coiling. Johns Hopkins Medicine. 2019. (https://www.hopkinsmedicine.org/health/treatment-tests-and-therapies/endovascular-coiling)

Lesions B. Causes, Symptoms, Treatments. WebMD. 2019. (https://www.webmd.com/brain/brain-lesions-causes-symptoms-treatments#1–4)

Vascular Malformations of the Brain. National Organization for Rare Disorders. 2006. (https://rarediseases.org/rare-diseases/vascular-malformations-of-the-brain/)

IV

# 10 Epidural Hematoma Evacuation/ Subdural Hematoma Evacuation/ Intracerebral Hemorrhage Evacuation

*Ryan F. Amidon, Christ Ordookhanian, and Paul E. Kaloostian*

## 10.1 Symptoms and Signs

- State of confusion
- Headache
- Vomiting or nausea
- Fatigue
- Difficulty producing speech
- Abnormal sleeping behavior
- Difficulty maintaining balance
- Blurred vision, abnormal taste/smell senses
- Mood change
- Memory or concentration deficiency
- Depression or anxiety
- Pupil dilation
- Weakness/numbness in fingers/toes
- Coma
- Neurologic dysfunction from cranial nerve damage

## 10.2 Surgical Pathology

- Cranial benign/malignant trauma

## 10.3 Diagnostic Modalities

- Physical examination
- Neurological examination
- Glasgow Coma Scale
- MRI of brain without contrast (see ▶ Fig. 10.1 and ▶ Fig. 10.2)
- CT scan of brain without contrast (see ▶ Fig. 10.3)
- X-ray of brain (test for skull fractures)

## 10.4 Differential Diagnosis

- Diffuse axonal injury (DAI)
- Concussion

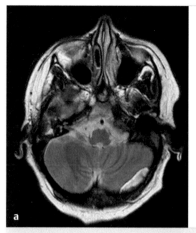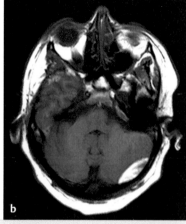

**Fig. 10.1** (a, b) MRI scans reveal left epidural hematoma located in the posterior cranial fossa 10 days after head trauma. (Source: Primary traumatic lesions. In: Forsting M, Jansen O, eds. MR Neuroimaging: Brain, Spine, Peripheral Nerves. 1st ed. Thieme; 2016).

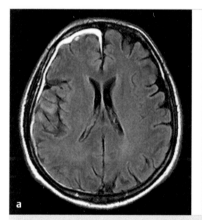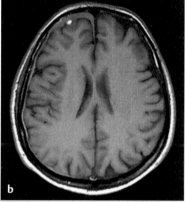

**Fig. 10.2** (a, b) MRI scans reveal right subdural hematoma and hemorrhagic contusion 8 days after head trauma. (Source: Primary traumatic lesions. In: Forsting M, Jansen O, eds. MR Neuroimaging: Brain, Spine, Peripheral Nerves. 1st ed. Thieme; 2016).

- Contusion
- Coup/Contrecoup lesion
- Skull fracture
- Hematoma
  - Epidural hematoma (bleeding between skull and dura mater)

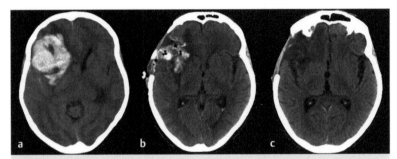

**Fig. 10.3** Preoperative CT scan revealed right frontal intracerebral hemorrhage in an elderly woman (**a**). After craniectomy and hematoma evacuation, postoperative CT revealed minimal damage to relevant brain tissue (**b**). Follow-up CT (6 weeks) demonstrates successful operation (**c**). (Source: Surgical management of spontaneous intracerebral hemorrhage. In: Nader R, Gragnanielldo C, Berta S, et al, eds. Neurosurgery Tricks of the Trade: Cranial. 1st ed. Thieme; 2013).

- – Subdural hematoma (bleeding between dura and arachnoid mater)
- – Subarachnoid hemorrhage (bleeding between arachnoid mater and pia mater)
- – Intracerebral hematoma (bleeding into brain itself)
- Degenerative brain disease from repeated or severe traumatic brain injury (TBI)
  - – Alzheimer's disease
  - – Parkinson's disease
  - – Dementia pugilistica

# 10.5 Treatment Options

- Acute pain control with medications and pain management
- Therapy and rehabilitation:
  - – Physiatry
  - – Occupational therapy
  - – Physical therapy
  - – Speech pathology
  - – Neuropsychology
  - – Rehabilitation nursing
  - – Recreational therapy
- If symptomatic:
  - – In emergent cases, ensure sufficient blood and oxygen supply
  - – Medications to reduce secondary damage (diuretics, antiseizure drugs, coma-inducing drugs)

- Surgery if deemed suitable candidate
  - Determine overall prognosis and Karnofsky performance score
  - If poor surgical candidate with poor life expectancy, medical management recommended
  - Hematoma removal
  - Skull fracture repair
  - Craniectomy (to relieve intracranial pressure and prevent herniation) followed by cranioplasty
  - Procedure with the intent to cease cerebral bleeding

## 10.6 Indications for Surgical Intervention

- No improvement after nonoperative therapy
- Neurologic dysfunction resulting from moderate to severe lesion
- Extensive brain swelling
- Damaged brain tissue
- Skull fracture
- Hematoma thicker than 10 mm with midline shift

## 10.7 Surgical Procedure for Subdural Hematoma/Epidural Hematoma/ Intraparenchymal Hematoma Evacuation

1. Informed consent signed, preoperative labs normal, patient ceases intaking of NSAIDs (Naprosyn, Advil, Nuprin, Motrin, Aleve) and blood thinners (Coumadin, Plavix, Aspirin) 1 week prior to treatment
2. Appropriate intubation and sedation and lines (if necessary) as per the anesthetist
3. Place patient in prone position on operating table, head flipped 90 degrees, and all pressure points padded
4. Neuromonitoring not needed
5. Time out is performed with agreement from everyone in the room for correct patient and correct surgery with consent signed
6. Perform skin incision over the level of hematoma, controlling superficial bleeding
7. Turn skin flap, using retractor
8. Expose scalp, using monopolar forceps
   a. Continue exposure
   b. Slightly move periosteum to side, using retractor
9. Drill burr holes into skull and perform craniotomy
   a. Move bone fragments aside to prevent infection

10. If epidural hematoma present, remove the clot at this point and stop arterial or venous bleeder with coagulation
11. Elevate and open the dura (a needle and thread approach, followed by scissors, may be used), exposing subdural hematoma
12. Perform hematoma evacuation:
    a. Carefully cut through any film covering hematoma
    b. Use suction to resect hematoma (do not let it touch the brain)
    c. If venous or arterial bleeding noted, this must be coagulated
13. If intraparenchymal hemorrhage present, must remove large superficial clot and coagulate bleeding with bipolar and Surgicel
14. Close the dura using sutures and duragen material
15. Re-implant bone flap, anchoring it with screws
16. Close skin incision in standard fashion

## 10.8 Pitfalls

- Neurologic deficits
- Recurrence of hematoma/hemorrhage
- Postoperative infection
- Postoperative seizure
- Emergence of contralateral hematoma
- Subdural empyema, brain abscess, and/or meningitis (when operative drainage is employed)

## 10.9 Prognosis

- Patient will be taken to a recovery room and ultimately to the intensive care unit (ICU). Hospitalization rates depend on the type of procedure performed, preoperative examination status, and patient's age/comorbidities.
- Headache, nausea, or vomiting, if present following the procedure, will warrant relevant medications

## Bibliography

Engelhard H. Subdural Hematoma Surgery. Medscape. 2018. (https://emedicine.medscape.com/article/247472-overview)

How Does TBI Affect the Brain? Brainline. 2019. (https://www.brainline.org/article/how-does-tbi-affect-brain)

Prinz V, Czabanka M. Acute Subdural Hematoma Evacuation. Journal of Medical Insight. (https://jomi.com/article/140/acute-subdural-hematoma-evacuation/procedure-outline)

Traumatic Brain Injury. Mayo Clinic. 2019. (https://www.mayoclinic.org/diseases-conditions/traumatic-brain-injury/symptoms-causes/syc-20378557)

# 11 Hemicraniectomy (Unilateral, Bilateral, Bifrontal versus Frontotemporal)

*Ryan F. Amidon, Christ Ordookhanian, and Paul E. Kaloostian*

## 11.1 Symptoms and Signs

- State of confusion
- Headache
- Vomiting or nausea
- Fatigue
- Difficulty producing speech
- Abnormal sleeping behavior
- Difficulty maintaining balance
- Blurred vision, abnormal taste/smell senses
- Mood change
- Memory or concentration deficiency
- Depression or anxiety
- Pupil dilation
- Weakness/Numbness in fingers/toes
- Coma
- Neurologic dysfunction from cranial nerve damage

## 11.2 Surgical Pathology

- Cranial benign/malignant trauma

## 11.3 Diagnostic Modalities

- Physical examination
- Neurological examination
- Glasgow Coma Scale
- CT scan of brain without contrast (see ▶ Fig. 11.1)
- MRI of brain without contrast
- X-ray of brain (test for skull fractures)

## 11.4 Differential Diagnosis

- Diffuse axonal injury (DAI)
- Concussion
- Contusion

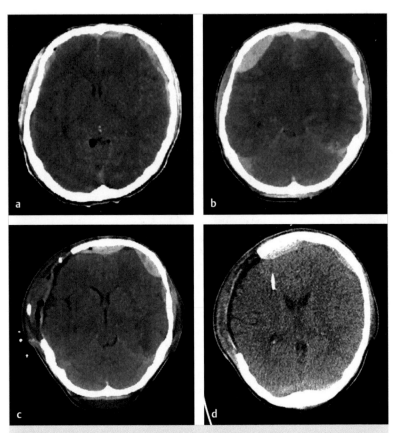

**Fig. 11.1** Preoperative CT scans revealed growing epidural right frontal hematoma in a young adult after suffering traumatic brain injury (TBI) (**a, b**). The patient received a right frontal craniotomy and hematoma evacuation (**c**) and a decompressive hemicraniectomy was performed to counteract increasing intracranial pressure (**d**). (Source: Westermaier T, Nickl R, Koehler S, et al. Selective brain cooling after traumatic brain injury: effects of three different cooling methods—case report. J Neurol Surg A Cent Eur Neurosurg 2017;78(4):397–402).

- Coup/Contrecoup lesion
- Skull fracture
- Hematoma
  - Epidural hematoma (bleeding between skull and dura mater) (see ▶Fig. 11.2)

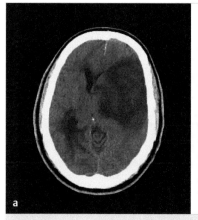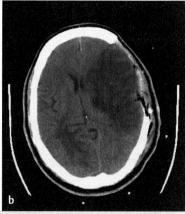

**Fig. 11.2** A CT scan was taken 1 week after left middle cerebral artery occlusive ischemic stroke (**a**). Symptoms of aphasia and left hemiplegia suggested subfalcine and uncal herniation. A left hemicraniectomy was performed (**b**). (Source: "Salvage" procedures for brain swelling post stroke. In: Loftus C, ed. Neurosurgical Emergencies. 3rd ed. Thieme; 2017).

- – Subdural hematoma (bleeding between dura and arachnoid mater)
- – Subarachnoid hemorrhage (bleeding between arachnoid mater and pia mater)
- – Intracerebral hematoma (bleeding into brain itself)
- Degenerative brain disease from repeated or severe traumatic brain injury (TBI)
  - – Alzheimer's disease
  - – Parkinson's disease
  - – Dementia pugilistica

## 11.5 Treatment Options

- Acute pain control with medications and pain management
- Therapy and rehabilitation
  - – Physiatry
  - – Occupational therapy
  - – Physical therapy
  - – Speech pathology
  - – Neuropsychology
  - – Rehabilitation nursing
  - – Recreational therapy

- If symptomatic:
  - In emergent cases, ensure sufficient blood and oxygen supply
  - Medications to reduce secondary damage (diuretics, antiseizure drugs, coma-inducing drugs)
  - Surgery if deemed suitable candidate
    - Determine overall prognosis and Karnofsky performance score
    - If poor surgical candidate with poor life expectancy, medical management recommended
    - Hematoma removal
    - Skull fracture repair
    - Hemicraniectomy (to relieve intracranial pressure and prevent herniation) followed by cranioplasty
      - Unilateral or bilateral
      - Bifrontal or frontotemporal
      - Unilateral frontotemporal: Unilateral localized lesion (traumatic hematoma and brain swelling from middle cerebral artery infarction)
      - Bifrontal: Frontal contusion of brain, generalized cerebral edema without localized lesion
    - Procedure with the intent to cease cerebral bleeding

## 11.6 Indications for Surgical Intervention

- No improvement after nonoperative therapy (medication, oxygen therapy, lowering body temperature)
- Damaged brain tissue
- Skull fracture
- Intracranial pressure compromising cerebral perfusion pressure and resulting in neurologic deterioration and brain herniations

## 11.7 Surgical Procedure for Unilateral Frontotemporoparietal Craniectomy

1. Informed consent signed, preoperative labs normal, patient ceases intaking of NSAIDs (Naprosyn, Advil, Nuprin, Motrin, Aleve) and blood thinners (Coumadin, Plavix, Aspirin) 1 week prior to treatment
2. Appropriate intubation and sedation and lines (if necessary) as per the anesthetist
3. Place patient in supine position on operating table, head turned to contralateral side (sagittal head angle 0 to 15 degrees horizontal to floor), and all pressure points padded
4. Neuromonitoring not needed

5. Time out is performed with agreement from everyone in the room for correct patient and correct surgery with consent signed
6. Perform "reverse question mark shape" incision from midline anterior to coronal suture, a few centimeters posterior to ear, and continue to root of zygoma
   a. Make incision 2 cm lateral to midline, preventing damage to superior sagittal sinus (SSS)
7. Create bone flap (over 15 cm in anteroposterior diameter), extending toward floor of temporal fossa for sufficient decompression
8. Drill four burr holes at the following points: temporal squama, parietal area posterior to parietal bone (near skin incision), frontal area 2 cm in front of coronal suture (near skin incision), and key hole region behind zygomatic arch of frontal bone
9. Achieve proper hemostasis
10. Close wound in standard fashion with stitches

# 11.8  Surgical Procedure for Bifrontal Craniectomy

1. Informed consent signed, preoperative labs normal, patient ceases intaking of NSAIDs (Naprosyn, Advil, Nuprin, Motrin, Aleve) and blood thinners (Coumadin, Plavix, Aspirin) 1 week prior to treatment
2. Appropriate intubation and sedation and lines (if necessary) as per the anesthetist
3. Place patient in supine position on operating table, all pressure points padded
4. Neuromonitoring not needed
5. Time out is performed with agreement from everyone in the room for correct patient and correct surgery with consent signed
6. Perform skin incision anterior to tragus on each side and curve cranially 2–3 cm posterior to coronal suture, continuing through galea and temporalis muscle to bone
   a. Ensure no damage to superficial temporal artery (STA)
7. Reflect the scalp and muscle flap forward over orbital rim, exposing both supraorbital nerves
8. Carefully dissect out supraorbital nerve from supraorbital notch bilaterally
   a. If supraorbital notch is closed, small osteotome can be made to open it
9. Create the following burr holes: Both key hole areas behind zygomatic arch of frontal bone, both squamous parts of temporal bones, two

holes just behind coronal suture (1 cm apart from midline on each side)
10. Dissect SSS away from bone flap by passing Penfield 3 between the burr holes
    a. Perform craniotomy over SSS with the last cut
11. After bone flap elevation, control bleeding from SSS using Gelfoam or Surgicel covered with cottonoid
12. Divide anterior portion of SSS and underlying falx (durotomy)
    a. Ligate the most anterior part of SSS with two heavy sutures and cut to cross anterior portion of SSS
13. Frontal lobectomy may be performed, if necessary, to diminish mass effect and swelling
14. Achieve proper hemostasis
15. Close wound in standard fashion with stitches

## 11.9 Pitfalls

- Neurologic deficits
- Postoperative infection
- Stroke
- Brain damage from oxygen deprivation
- Extensive brain bleeding
- Subdural empyema, brain abscess, and/or meningitis (when operative drainage is employed)
- Damage to SSS
- Damage to tragus
- Worsening of brain herniation and future brain damage from inadequate decompression
- Damage to STA
- Damage to supraorbital nerves
- Cerebrospinal fluid (CSF) absorption disorder (subdural hygroma and hydrocephalus) and leakage
- Postoperative hematoma expansion
- Syndrome of the trephined

## 11.10 Prognosis

- Patient will be taken to a recovery room and ultimately to the ICU. Hospitalization rates depend on the type of procedure performed, preoperative examination status, and patient's age/comorbidities.

- Physical, speech, and/or exercise therapy may be necessary
- Headache, nausea, or vomiting, if present following the procedure, will warrant relevant medications
- Once patient is adequately recovered after surgery, a cranioplasty will be performed to replace missing portion of skull with original bone or titanium/synthetic bone

## Bibliography

Moon JW, Hyun DK. Decompressive craniectomy in traumatic brain injury: a review article. Korean J Neurotrauma. 2017; 13(1):1–8

Zawn V, Han S. What is a decompressive craniectomy? MedicalNewsToday. 2017. (https://www.medicalnewstoday.com/articles/319755.php)

# 12 Cranioplasty

*Ryan F. Amidon, Christ Ordookhanian, and Paul E. Kaloostian*

## 12.1 Symptoms and Signs

- State of confusion
- Headache
- Vomiting or nausea
- Fatigue
- Difficulty producing speech
- Abnormal sleeping behavior
- Difficulty maintaining balance
- Blurred vision, abnormal taste/smell senses
- Mood change
- Memory or concentration deficiency
- Depression or anxiety
- Pupil dilation
- Weakness/Numbness in fingers/toes
- Coma
- Neurologic dysfunction from cranial nerve damage

## 12.2 Surgical Pathology

- Cranial benign/malignant trauma

## 12.3 Diagnostic Modalities

- Physical examination
- Neurological examination
- Glasgow Coma Scale
- CT scan of brain without contrast (see ▶ Fig. 12.1)
- MRI of brain without contrast
- X-ray of brain (test for skull fractures)

## 12.4 Differential Diagnosis

- Diffuse axonal injury (DAI)
- Concussion
- Contusion
- Coup/Contrecoup lesion

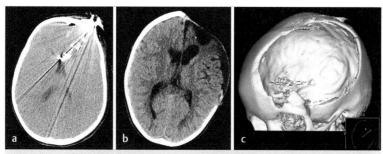

**Fig. 12.1** Preoperative CT scan revealed intracranial trauma and trajectory of left frontal gunshot wound in a 4-year-old child **(a)**. Decompression and superficial fragment evacuation were performed via cranioplasty **(b)**. Follow-up three-dimensional computed tomography (3D-CT; 6 months) **(c)**. (Source: Operative detail and preparation. In: Cohen A, ed. Pediatric Neurosurgery. 1st ed. Thieme; 2015).

- Skull fracture
- Hematoma
  - Epidural hematoma (bleeding between skull and dura mater)
  - Subdural hematoma (bleeding between dura and arachnoid mater)
  - Subarachnoid hemorrhage (bleeding between arachnoid mater and pia mater)
  - Intracerebral hematoma (bleeding into brain itself)
- Degenerative brain disease from repeated or severe traumatic brain injury (TBI)
  - Alzheimer's disease
  - Parkinson's disease
  - Dementia pugilistica

# 12.5 Treatment Options

## 12.5.1 Acute Pain Control with Medications and Pain Management

## 12.5.2 Therapy and Rehabilitation

- Physiatry
- Occupational therapy
- Physical therapy
- Speech pathology
- Neuropsychology
- Rehabilitation nursing
- Recreational therapy

### 12.5.3 If Symptomatic

- In emergent cases, ensure sufficient blood and oxygen supply
- Medications to reduce secondary damage (diuretics, antiseizure drugs, coma-inducing drugs)
- Surgery if deemed suitable candidate
  - Determine overall prognosis and Karnofsky performance score
  - If poor surgical candidate with poor life expectancy, medical management recommended
  - Hematoma removal
  - Skull fracture repair
  - Craniectomy (to relieve intracranial pressure and prevent herniation) followed by cranioplasty
- Unilateral or bilateral
- Bifrontal or frontotemporal
- Unilateral frontotemporal: Unilateral localized lesion (traumatic hematoma and brain swelling from middle cerebral artery infarction)
- Bifrontal: Frontal contusion of brain, generalized cerebral edema without localized lesion
  - Procedure with the intent to cease cerebral bleeding

## 12.6 Indications for Surgical Intervention

- No improvement after nonoperative therapy (medication, oxygen therapy, lowering body temperature)
- Severe headaches
- Neurological impairment
- Skull fracture
- To restore missing bone space after a craniectomy is performed to reduce intracranial pressure
- Abnormal skull shape
- Brain tissue vulnerable to damage

## 12.7 Surgical Procedure for Cranioplasty

1. Informed consent signed, preoperative labs normal, patient ceases intaking of NSAIDs (Naprosyn, Advil, Nuprin, Motrin, Aleve) and blood thinners (Coumadin, Plavix, Aspirin) 1 week prior to treatment
2. Appropriate intubation and sedation and lines (if necessary) as per the anesthetist
3. Place patient in appropriate position to reach the skull locus on operating table, with all pressure points padded
4. Neuromonitoring not needed

5. Time out is performed with agreement from everyone in the room for correct patient and correct surgery with consent signed
6. Shave and clean area of incision with antiseptic solution
7. Perform incision in scalp over prior incision
   a. Carefully dissect skin into layers, protecting the dura
8. Clean edges of surrounding bone
9. Prepare surface so that bone or implant can be properly positioned in defect
10. Insert bone or implant into the defect, attaching it to nearby bones via titanium plates and screws
    a. Bone grafts from rib, skull, or pelvis
    b. Titanium or synthetic bone
    c. Acrylic inserts
11. Achieve proper hemostasis
12. Return scalp to original position
13. Close skin incision with nylon suture

# 12.8 Pitfalls

- Neurologic deficits
- Postoperative infection
- Blood clot formation (requires drainage)
- Postoperative seizures
- Stroke

# 12.9 Prognosis

- Patient will be taken to a recovery room and ultimately to the neurosurgical floor or neurological critical care unit (NCCU). Hospitalization rates depend on the type of procedure performed, preoperative examination status, and patient's age/comorbidities (normally 2–7 days).
- Drain may be placed to remove excess fluid accumulated in brain (removed in several days)
- Headache, nausea, or vomiting, if present following the procedure, will warrant relevant medications

# Bibliography

Cranioplasty. Johns Hopkins Medicine. (https://www.hopkinsmedicine.org/health/treatment-tests-and-therapies/cranioplasty)

Cranioplasty. Princeton Neurological Surgery. (http://www.princetonneurologicalsurgery.com/our-services/brain-surgery/cranioplasty/)

# 13 Placement of External Ventricular Drain/Placement of Intraparenchymal ICP Monitor

*Ryan F. Amidon, Christ Ordookhanian, and Paul E. Kaloostian*

## 13.1 Symptoms and Signs

- State of confusion
- Headache
- Vomiting or nausea
- Fatigue
- Difficulty producing speech
- Abnormal sleeping behavior
- Difficulty maintaining balance
- Blurred vision, abnormal taste/smell senses
- Mood change
- Memory or concentration deficiency
- Depression or anxiety
- Pupil dilation
- Weakness/Numbness in fingers/toes
- Coma
- Neurologic dysfunction from cranial nerve damage

## 13.2 Surgical Pathology

- Cranial benign/malignant trauma

## 13.3 Diagnostic Modalities

- Physical examination
- Neurological examination
- Glasgow Coma Scale
- CT scan of brain without contrast
- MRI of brain without contrast
- X-ray of brain (test for skull fractures)

## 13.4 Differential Diagnosis

- Diffuse axonal injury (DAI)
- Concussion

- Contusion
- Coup/Contrecoup lesion
- Skull fracture
- Hematoma
  - Epidural hematoma (bleeding between skull and dura mater)
  - Subdural hematoma (bleeding between dura and arachnoid mater)
  - Subarachnoid hemorrhage (bleeding between arachnoid mater and pia mater)
  - Intracerebral hematoma (bleeding into brain itself)
- Degenerative brain disease from repeated or severe traumatic brain injury (TBI)
  - Alzheimer's disease
  - Parkinson's disease
  - Dementia pugilistica

## 13.5  Treatment Options

### 13.5.1  Acute Pain Control with Medications and Pain Management

### 13.5.2  Therapy and Rehabilitation

- Physiatry
- Occupational therapy
- Physical therapy
- Speech pathology
- Neuropsychology
- Rehabilitation nursing
- Recreational therapy

### 13.5.3  If Symptomatic

- In emergent cases, ensure sufficient blood and oxygen supply
- Medications to reduce secondary damage (diuretics, antiseizure drugs, coma-inducing drugs)
- Surgery if deemed suitable candidate
  - Determine overall prognosis and Karnofsky performance score
  - If poor surgical candidate with poor life expectancy, medical management recommended
  - Hematoma removal
  - Skull fracture repair

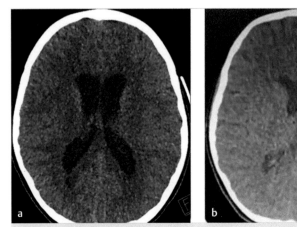

**Fig. 13.1** Before placement of external ventricular drain (EVD), intracranial pressure (ICP) was elevated, cerebrospinal fluid (CSF) leakage was present, and the ventricles were enlarged (**a**). Postplacement imaging confirms success of EVD effect (**b**). (Source: Adjuncts and postoperative care. In: Stamm A, ed. Transnasal Endoscopic Skull Base and Brain Surgery: Surgical Anatomy and Its Applications. 2nd ed. Thieme; 2019).

- External ventricular drain (EVD) placement to treat hydrocephalus and reduce elevated intracranial pressure (ICP), when normal cerebrospinal fluid (CSF) flow is obstructed or intracranial swelling is noted (see ►Fig. 13.1)
- Intraparenchymal ICP monitor placement to measure ICP without CSF diversion
- Craniectomy (to relieve ICP and prevent herniation) followed by cranioplasty
  - Unilateral or bilateral
  - Bifrontal or frontotemporal
  - Unilateral frontotemporal: Unilateral localized lesion (traumatic hematoma and cerebral swelling)
  - Bifrontal: Frontal contusion of brain, generalized cerebral edema without localized lesion

## 13.6 Indications for Surgical Intervention

- No improvement after nonoperative therapy (medication, oxygen therapy, lowering body temperature)
- Severe headaches

- Neurological impairment
- Elevated ICP
- Need to record ICP
- Hydrocephalus
- Normal CSF flow obstructed or cerebral swelling noted (EVD placement procedure)
- No need to divert CSF flow (intraparenchymal ICP monitor placement procedure)
- Intraventricular hemorrhage

# 13.7  Surgical Procedure for EVD Placement

1. Informed consent signed, preoperative labs normal, patient ceases intaking of NSAIDs (Naprosyn, Advil, Nuprin, Motrin, Aleve) and blood thinners (Coumadin, Plavix, Aspirin) 1 week prior to treatment
2. Appropriate intubation and sedation and lines (if necessary) as per the anesthetist
3. Place patient in supine position on operating table, head of bed elevated at 45 degrees, and all pressure points padded
4. Neuromonitoring not needed
5. Time out is performed with agreement from everyone in the room for correct patient and correct surgery with consent signed
6. Shave and clean area of incision with antiseptic solution
   a. Right frontal cerebral hemisphere preferred site of entry due to its nondominance for language function in over 90% of patients
7. Create incision in scalp, properly exposing skull
8. Create burr hole at Kocher's point, avoiding superior sagittal sinus (SSS) and frontal cortex motor strip
   a. Locate this point by drawing one line in midline from nasion to a point 10 cm back and another from the previous point to a site 3 cm lateral to it, along ipsilateral midpupillary line
9. Perform linear skin incision down to bone and scrape the periosteum
10. Penetrate cranium using twist drill, in trajectory determined for ventricular cannulation (craniostomy)
11. Pierce pia and dura with scalpel
12. Prime ventricular catheter and pass it no more than 7 mm, aiming in a coronal plane toward medical canthus of ipsilateral eye and in the anteroposterior plane toward a point 1.5 cm anterior to ipsilateral tragus, toward ipsilateral Foramen of Monro
13. Visualize CSF flow after removing catheter stylet and transduce it to obtain opening for ICP

14. Tunnel catheter through skin away from point of entry through separate incision, sutured securely in place (with staples to fixate catheter to scalp), and then connected to external drainage system
15. EVD placement is complete

# 13.8 Surgical Procedure for Intraparenchymal ICP Monitor Placement

1. Informed consent signed, preoperative labs normal, patient ceases intaking of NSAIDs (Naprosyn, Advil, Nuprin, Motrin, Aleve) and blood thinners (Coumadin, Plavix, Aspirin) 1 week prior to treatment
2. Appropriate intubation and sedation and lines (if necessary) as per the anesthetist
3. Place patient in supine position on operating table, head of bed elevated at 45 degrees, and all pressure points padded
4. Neuromonitoring not needed
5. Time out is performed with agreement from everyone in the room for correct patient and correct surgery with consent signed
6. Shave and clean area of incision with antiseptic solution
   a. Right or left prefrontal area preferred for intraparenchymal ICP monitor placement (right hemisphere more common) (see ▶ Fig. 13.2)
7. Make an incision in scalp, 2–3 cm anterior to coronal suture in a plate with midpupillary line behind hairline
8. Perform 0.5 cm linear incision down to bone

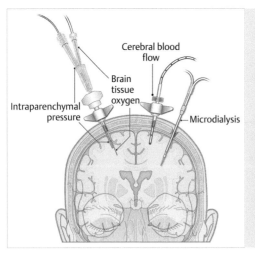

**Fig. 13.2** Illustrative guide to placement of intraparenchymal intracranial pressure (ICP) monitor. It is placed no more than 2.5 cm deep to measure ICP and is secured to a bolt system or the skin. Image also provides positioning of brain tissue oxygen monitors, cerebral blood flow monitors, and microdialysis catheters. (Source: Operative procedure. In: Ullman J, Raksin P, eds. Atlas of Emergency Neurosurgery. 1st ed. Thieme; 2015).

Cerebral blood flow

Brain tissue oxygen

Intraparenchymal pressure

Microdialysis

9. Expose bone using small skin retractor and achieve hemostasis of skin edges
10. Drill twist drill hole through outer and inner tables of skull
    a. Do not penetrate dura or brain (ensure drill guard is in place)
11. Remove drill and irrigate with sterile saline
12. Puncture dura with spinal needle
13. Screw bolt into skull manually
14. Insert stylet through the bolt to remove bone or soft tissue debris
15. Attach fiberoptic catheter to monitor
    a. Adjust monitor to calibrate fiberoptic cable to "zero" (if necessary)
16. Insert fiberoptic catheter through strain-relief protective sheath and then into bolt, so that it extends 0.5 cm beyond end of bolt into parenchyma
17. Pull back on catheter 1 to 2 mm so that it is not under tension against blood vessel or parenchyma
18. Turn compression cap clockwise to secure monitor in place
19. Place Tegaderm, securing strain-relief protective sheath to fiberoptic cable
20. Check for pressure waveform and record initial ICP
21. Interpret waveforms (i.e., A, B, and C waves)

# 13.9 Pitfalls

- Neurologic deficits
- Postoperative infection
- Hemorrhage
- Inadvertent placement into brain tissue
- CSF obstruction

# 13.10 Prognosis

- Hospitalization rates depend on the type of procedure performed, preoperative examination status, and patient's age/comorbidities
- Management and surveillance of EVD or intraparenchymal ICP monitor will continue
- Headache, nausea, or vomiting, if present following the procedure, will warrant relevant medications

# Bibliography

Gupta G, Roychowdhury S, Nosko M. Intracranial Pressure Monitoring Technique. Medscape. 2018. (https://emedicine.medscape.com/article/1829950-technique)
Muralidharan R. External ventricular drains: management and complications. Surg Neurol Int. 2015; 6(Suppl 6):S271–S274

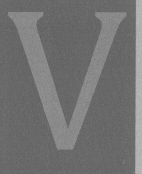

# 14 Deep Brain Stimulation

*Ryan F. Amidon, Christ Ordookhanian, and Paul E. Kaloostian*

## 14.1 Symptoms and Signs

- Chronic headaches
- Difficulty in movement
- Memory or concentration deficiency
- Depression or anxiety
- Behavioral tics
- Seizures
- Memory deficiency

## 14.2 Surgical Pathology

- Cranial benign/malignant movement disorder
- Cranial benign/malignant psychiatric condition
- Cranial benign/malignant trauma

## 14.3 Diagnostic Modalities

- Physical examination
- Neurological examination
- PET scan of brain
- CT scan of brain
- MRI of brain

## 14.4 Differential Diagnosis

- Movement disorders
  - Dystonia
  - Parkinson's disease
  - Essential tremor
- Psychiatric conditions (still under study)
  - Obsessive-compulsive disorder
  - Depression (major)
  - Addiction
  - Dementia
  - Schizophrenia
- Huntington's disease (still under study)
- Multiple sclerosis (still under study)

- Tourette syndrome (still under study)
- Stroke recovery (still under study)
- Traumatic brain injury (TBI) (still under study)

## 14.5 Treatment Options

- Acute pain control with medications and pain management
- Therapy and rehabilitation
  - Physiatry
  - Occupational therapy
  - Physical therapy
  - Speech pathology
  - Neuropsychology
  - Rehabilitation nursing
  - Recreational therapy
- If symptomatic and no improvement after nonoperative management:
  - Deep brain stimulation (implanting electrodes in brain to regulate abnormal impulses and brain activity)
    - Amount of stimulation controlled by pacemaker-like device under skin in upper chest (a subcutaneous wire connects this device to electrodes in brain)

## 14.6 Indications for Surgical Intervention

- No improvement after nonoperative therapy such as medication treatments
- Severe, chronic headaches
- Neurological impairment
- Difficult-to-treat epilepsy
- Advanced symptoms of movement and/or psychiatric disorder(s)

## 14.7 Surgical Procedure for Deep Brain Stimulation

1. Informed consent signed, preoperative labs normal, patient ceases intaking of NSAIDs (Naprosyn, Advil, Nuprin, Motrin, Aleve) and blood thinners (Coumadin, Plavix, Aspirin) 1 week prior to treatment
2. Appropriate intubation and sedation and lines (if necessary) as per the anesthetist
   a. Procedure can be accomplished without general anesthesia, requiring local anesthesia to numb scalp before procedure
3. Place patient in supine position for stimulation on operating table, with Mayfield Pin fixation, and all pressure points padded

4. Neuromonitoring is needed during awake testing portion of the procedure with neurological evaluation
5. Time out is performed with agreement from everyone in the room for correct patient and correct surgery with consent signed
6. Shave (if necessary) and clean area of incision with antiseptic solution
7. Make an incision in scalp, properly exposing skull
8. Create small opening in skull and insert lead (electrode) through brain and implant in predetermined locus with a number of contacts, under computerized imaging stereotactic guidance (see ▶ Fig. 14.1 and ▶ Fig. 14.2)
9. Implant internal pulse generator (IPG)
   a. Place patient under general anesthesia

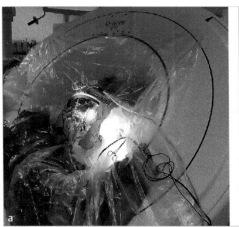
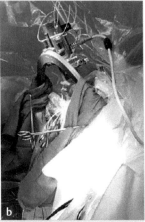

**Fig. 14.1** (a, b) Stanford frame-based setup for deep brain stimulation (DBS) lead placement. An O-arm intraoperative CT scanner and microelectrode recording hardware are present. (Source: Surgical flow and DBS lead placement. In: Anderson W, ed. Deep Brain Stimulation: Techniques and Practices. 1st ed. Thieme; 2019).

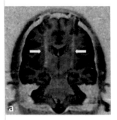
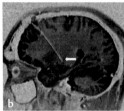

**Fig. 14.2** (a, b) MRI scans confirm deep brain stimulation (DBS) lead placement bilaterally in the subthalamic nucleus. (Source: Postoperative imaging. In: Kanekar S, ed. Imaging of Neurodegenerative Disorders. 1st ed. Thieme; 2015).

b. Implant part of IPG containing the batteries (pulse generator) under skin in chest, near collarbone (it may also be implanted in chest or under skin over abdomen)

10. Connect electrodes via wires to IPG
    a. An extension wire is passed under skin of head, neck, and shoulder to the IPG
    b. Magnet is used with IPG to adjust stimulation parameters
    c. IPG may be turned on or off using a remote control

# 14.8 Pitfalls

- Postoperative infection
- Stroke
- Extensive brain bleeding
- Misplacement of lead (electrode) or lead wire erosion
- Breathing abnormalities
- Heart problems
- Postoperative seizure
- Nausea/Confusion
- Speech, balance, and/or visual deficiencies
- Undesirable mood changes
- Undesirable sensory changes
- Muscle tightness of face or arm

# 14.9 Prognosis

- Hospitalization rates depend on the type of procedure performed, preoperative examination status, and patient's age/comorbidities
- Pulse generator in chest activated by physician a few weeks after surgery
  - It may take months to find optimal setting for one's specific condition
- Headache, nausea, or vomiting, if present following the procedure, will warrant relevant medications
- IPG batteries last 3 to 5 years and will need to be replaced under local anesthesia as an outpatient procedure

# Bibliography

Deep Brain Stimulation. American Association of Neurological Surgeons. 2019. (https://www.aans.org/Patients/Neurosurgical-Conditions-and-Treatments/Deep-Brain-Stimulation)

Deep Brain Stimulation. Mayo Clinic. 2018. (https://www.mayoclinic.org/tests-procedures/deep-brain-stimulation/about/pac-20384562)

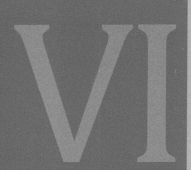

# Section VI

**Epilepsy**

# 15 Subdural Grid Placement

*Ryan F. Amidon, Christ Ordookhanian, and Paul E. Kaloostian*

## 15.1 Symptoms and Signs

- Seizures
- Temporary confusion
- Staring spell
- Loss of consciousness/awareness
- Fear, anxiety, or deja vu

## 15.2 Surgical Pathology

- Cranial benign/malignant neurological disorder
- Cranial benign/malignant trauma
- Cranial benign/malignant developmental disorder

## 15.3 Diagnostic Modalities

- Physical examination
- Neurological examination
- Blood test
- Electroencephalogram (EEG) of brain
- High-density EEG of brain
- PET scan of brain
- CT scan of brain
- MRI of brain
- Functional MRI (fMRI) of brain
- Statistical parametric mapping (SPM) of brain
- Curry analysis
- Magnetoencephalography (MEG) of brain
- Single photon emission computed tomography (SPECT) of brain
- Grid and strip electrode placement
  - Strips: 1 × 4 to 2 × 8 electrodes
  - Grids: 4 × 4 to 8 × 8 electrodes (16 to 64 contacts, respectively)
  - Contacts typically spaced 5 to 10 mm apart

## 15.4 Differential Diagnosis

- Generalized seizure
  - Absence seizure (petit mal; brief loss of awareness)
  - Tonic seizure (muscle stiffening, falling)

- Atonic seizure (loss of muscle control, collapse)
- Clonic seizure (repeated jerking muscle movements)
- Myoclonic seizure (sudden brief jerks of arms and legs)
- Tonic-clonic seizure (grand mal; abrupt loss of consciousness, body stiffening and shaking, loss of bladder control, biting of tongue)
- Focal seizure
  - Without loss of consciousness (alter emotions or change perception of environment, involuntary jerking of body part, spontaneous sensory tingling, dizziness, and flashing lights)
  - With impaired awareness (staring into space, performing repetitive movements like hand rubbing or walking in circles)

## 15.5 Treatment Options

- Antiepileptic medication
- Therapy and rehabilitation
  - Physiatry
  - Occupational therapy
  - Physical therapy
  - Speech pathology
  - Neuropsychology
  - Rehabilitation nursing
  - Recreational therapy
  - Vagus nerve stimulation
  - Ketogenic diet
- If symptomatic and no improvement after nonoperative management:
  - Epilepsy surgery
  - Deep brain stimulation (implanting electrodes in brain to regulate abnormal impulses and brain activity)
    - Amount of stimulation controlled by pacemaker-like device under skin in upper chest (a subcutaneous wire connects this device to electrodes in brain)

## 15.6 Indications for Surgical Intervention

- Difficult-to-treat epilepsy
- Work-up of medically refractory partial epilepsy (focal seizures)
- All noninvasive diagnostic options for localization of epileptogenic zone exhausted
- Dual pathology, nonlesional epilepsy, extratemporal epilepsy, or lateral temporal lobe epilepsy implicated

# 15.7 Surgical Procedure for Subdural Grid Placement

1. Informed consent signed, preoperative labs normal, patient ceases intaking of NSAIDs (Naprosyn, Advil, Nuprin, Motrin, Aleve) and blood thinners (Coumadin, Plavix, Aspirin) 1 week prior to treatment
2. Appropriate intubation and sedation and lines (if necessary) as per the anesthetist
3. Place patient in supine position for stimulation on operating table, with Mayfield Pin fixation, and all pressure points padded
4. Neuromonitoring may be required to monitor nerves (if necessary and indicated)
5. Time out is performed with agreement from everyone in the room for correct patient and correct surgery with consent signed
6. Shave entire head and clean with antiseptic solution
7. Perform craniotomy (location determined based on preoperative studies)
   a. Access to large areas of head facilitated by skull clamp
   b. Make skin incision around appropriate skull region
   c. Turn skin flap, using retractor
   d. Expose scalp, using monopolar forceps
   e. Drill burr holes into skull
   f. Elevate a large C-shaped trauma and craniotomy flap
   g. Ensure protection of superficial temporal artery (STA) to preserve vascularity to the scalp flap
8. Establish grid within subdural space (see ▶ Fig. 15.1)
   a. Slide electrode underneath edges of craniotomy, gently injecting irrigation fluid, allowing grid to slide through more easily toward destination
   b. If necessary, cut or trim grid arrays to further conform to cortical surface
   c. Stay clear of parasagittal bridging veins
   d. Slits may be made in rows at the periphery of grid to taper edges, allowing good fit along boundaries of dural opening
   e. e. If placing double-sided grid electrodes within interhemispheric space:
      i. Remove bone over superior sagittal sinus (SSS) and open the dura, carefully avoiding the bridging veins
   f. Space grid contacts 5 to 10 mm apart in loci suspected to influence epileptic activity, as determined from preoperative studies
9. Perform electrode wire tunneling
   a. Insert multiple angiocaths (10 GA, 3.4 mm, 3 in) through separate stab incisions about an inch from skin edge, in order to tunnel the wires percutaneously

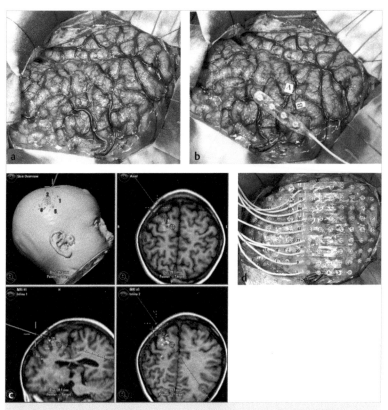

**Fig. 15.1** **(a)** Initial view of right cerebral hemisphere for intractable rolandic epilepsy, following a craniotomy. **(b)** The central sulcus is identified by measuring inversion polarity. A labels magnetoencephalography (MEG) somatically evoked field (SEF) and B labels MEG monitor. **(c)** Frameless stereotaxy is employed to verify location of SEF based on preoperative MEG. In a three-dimensional reconstruction, the MEG spike cluster (pink) is within the desired subdural grid placement (blue). **(d)** Subdural grid, strips, and depth electrode placements are performed. Letters correspond to MEG clusters. (Source: Operative detail and preparation. In: Cohen A, ed. Pediatric Neurosurgery. 1st ed. Thieme; 2015).

b. Insert purse-string stitches around the wires to prevent cerebrospinal fluid (CSF) leakage from tracking along wires (to be removed during second operation of electrode explant and resection)
c. Tag and register the exiting wires corresponding to each electrode

10. Perform intraoperative skull X-ray photograph
11. Prepare color photographs and sketches and record location of electrodes in relation to major lobes and fissures/sulci
12. Confirm sufficient recording from implanted electrodes
13. Suture the electrodes along their borders to edges of dura, avoiding displacement during monitoring period
14. Complete duroplasty using segments of previously harvested pericranial autograft
15. Close dura in relatively watertight fashion
16. Place temporary epidural drain
17. Close scalp in two layers and use nylon sutures to approximate the skin

## 15.8  Pitfalls

- Neurologic damage
- Postoperative infection
- CSF leakage
- Electrode displacement
- Altered mental status
- Blood vessel damage

## 15.9  Prognosis

- Hospitalization rates depend on the type of procedure performed, preoperative examination status, and patient's age/comorbidities
- Epidural drain removed on first postoperative day after head CT is completed
- Bone flap will be replaced during second operation when electrodes are explanted and resection is conducted
- Headache, nausea, or vomiting, if present following the procedure, will warrant relevant medications

## Bibliography

Epilepsy. Mayo Clinic. 2019. (https://www.mayoclinic.org/diseases-conditions/epilepsy/symptoms-causes/syc-20350093)

Voorhies JM, Cohen-Gadol A. Techniques for placement of grid and strip electrodes for intracranial epilepsy surgery monitoring: pearls and pitfalls. Surg Neurol Int. 2013; 4:98

# 16 Amygdalohippocampectomy

*Ryan F. Amidon, Christ Ordookhanian, and Paul E. Kaloostian*

## 16.1 Symptoms and Signs

- Seizures
- Temporary confusion
- Staring spell
- Loss of consciousness/awareness
- Fear, anxiety, or deja vu

## 16.2 Surgical Pathology

- Cranial benign/malignant neurological disorder
- Cranial benign/malignant trauma
- Cranial benign/malignant developmental disorder

## 16.3 Diagnostic Modalities

- Physical examination
- Neurological examination
- Blood test
- Electroencephalogram (EEG) of brain
- High-density EEG of brain
- PET scan of brain
- CT scan of brain (see ▶ Fig. 16.1)
- MRI of brain
- Functional MRI (fMRI) of brain
- Statistical parametric mapping (SPM) of brain
- Curry analysis
- Magnetoencephalography (MEG) of brain
- Single photon emission computed tomography (SPECT) of brain
- Grid and strip electrode placement
  - Strips: 1 × 4 to 2 × 8 electrodes
  - Grids: 4 × 4 to 8 × 8 electrodes (16 to 64 contacts, respectively)

## 16.4 Differential Diagnosis

- Generalized seizure
  - Absence seizure (petit mal; brief loss of awareness)
  - Tonic seizure (muscle stiffening, falling)
  - Atonic seizure (loss of muscle control, collapse)

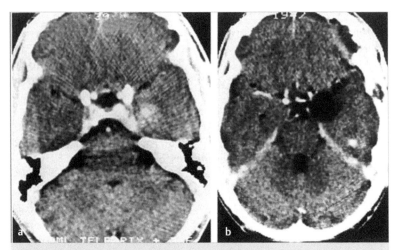

**Fig. 16.1** Preoperative CT scan revealed right amygdalohippocampal lesion (a cavernoma) in a middle-aged patient with temporal lobe seizures (**a**). The cavernoma was removed via a pterional approach and an amygdalohippocampectomy was performed (**b**). (Source: Clinical features and surgical results. In: Yasargil M, Curcic M, Teddy P, et al, eds. Microneurosurgery, Vol. III B. AVM of the Brain, Clinical Considerations, General and Special Operative Techniques, Surgical Results, Nonoperated Cases, Cavernous and Venous Angiomas, Neuroanesthesia. 1st ed. Thieme; 1998).

- Clonic seizure (repeated jerking muscle movements)
- Myoclonic seizure (sudden brief jerks of arms and legs)
- Tonic-clonic seizure (grand mal; abrupt loss of consciousness, body stiffening and shaking, loss of bladder control, biting of tongue)
- Focal seizure
  - Without loss of consciousness (alter emotions or change perception of environment, involuntary jerking of body part, spontaneous sensory tingling, dizziness, and flashing lights)
  - With impaired awareness (staring into space, performing repetitive movements like hand rubbing or walking in circles)

# 16.5 Treatment Options

## 16.5.1 Antiepileptic Medication (Neurological Evaluation)

## 16.5.2 Therapy and Rehabilitation

- Physiatry
- Occupational therapy

- Physical therapy
- Speech pathology
- Neuropsychology
- Rehabilitation nursing
- Recreational therapy
- Vagus nerve stimulation
- Ketogenic diet

## 16.5.3  If Symptomatic and No Improvement after Nonoperative Management

- Epilepsy surgery
  - Amygdalohippocampectomy (treats seizures from temporal lobe epilepsy beginning in medial-basal temporal lobe structures—hippocampus, amygdala, and parahippocampal gyrus)
    - Subtemporal approach (avoids Meyer loop injury, but may result in vein of Labbe injury)
    - Transcortical approach
    - Transsylvian approach (saves lateral temporal lobe)
- Deep brain stimulation (implanting electrodes in brain to regulate abnormal impulses and brain activity)
  - Amount of stimulation controlled by pacemaker-like device under skin in upper chest (a subcutaneous wire connects this device to electrodes in brain)

## 16.6  Indications for Surgical Intervention

- No improvement after nonoperative therapy
- Neurological impairment
- Difficult-to-treat epilepsy
- MRI demonstrates abnormality in mesial temporal structures
- Combatable ictal semiology and neurologic history
- EEG consistent with mesial temporal origin

## 16.7  Surgical Procedure for Transcortical Selective Amygdalohippocampectomy (SAH)

1. Informed consent signed, preoperative labs normal, patient ceases intaking of NSAIDs (Naprosyn, Advil, Nuprin, Motrin, Aleve) and blood thinners (Coumadin, Plavix, Aspirin) 1 week prior to treatment
2. Appropriate intubation and sedation and lines (if necessary) as per the anesthetist

3. Place patient in supine position on operating table, with Mayfield Pin fixation, head turned 90 degrees to contralateral side, and all pressure points padded
4. Neuromonitoring may be required to monitor nerves (if necessary and indicated)
5. Time out is performed with agreement from everyone in the room for correct patient and correct surgery with consent signed
6. Shave (if necessary) and clean site of incision with antiseptic solution
7. Perform scalp and temporalis fascia incision and retraction at appropriate locus
8. Perform craniotomy (location determined based on neuronavigation system):
   a. Drill burr holes into skull
   b. Elevate bone flap and open the dura
   c. Flap the dura inferiorly
9. Perform corticectomy:
   a. Identify location of cortical incision in middle temporal gyrus that is 2.5 to 3.0 cm behind tip of temporal lobe and in area free of cortical vessels, using neuronavigation system
   b. Perform corticectomy typically 2 to 2.5 cm in length
   c. Dissect toward temporal horn until temporal horn is entered
   d. Place two self-retaining brain retractors to visualize intraventricular anatomy, identifying key anatomical structures
   e. Resect parahippocampal gyrus, beginning with subpial resection of uncus and advancing medially and posteriorly
      i. Carefully preserve mesial pial border
   f. Visualize incisura as well as internal carotid artery and third nerve through the pia
   g. Identify choroidal fissure and ensure no dissection takes place superior to it
   h. Mobilize hippocampus laterally and resect beginning anteriorly, with care to preserve anterior choroidal artery, and carried posteriorly to the level of tectal plate
   i. After successful hippocampal resection, visualize cerebral peduncle and anterior choroidal artery through pia
   j. Confirm completeness of resection via neuronavigation
   k. Achieve proper hemostasis
10. Perform wound closure:
    a. Close dura
    b. Plate the bone flap
    c. Reapproximate temporalis muscle
    d. Close scalp in layers and use nylon sutures to approximate the skin

# 16.8 Pitfalls

- Neurologic damage
- Postoperative infection
- Cerebral vasospasm
- Visual field defects
- Hemorrhage
- Infarction (typically of deep penetrating vessels, resulting in lacunar stroke)
- Inaccurate or incomplete resection
- Meyer loop injury (typically asymptomatic)
- Memory deficiency
- Mood changes
- Blood vessel damage

# 16.9 Prognosis

- Overnight stay in neurological intensive care unit. Hospitalization rates depend on the type of procedure performed, preoperative examination status, and patient's age/comorbidities (typically 3–4 days)
- Postoperative neurological examination and head CT will be performed
- Continued antiepileptic medication will be prescribed
- Headache, nausea, or vomiting, if present following the procedure, will warrant relevant medications

# Bibliography

Amygdalohippocampectomy. Brain Recovery Project. (https://www.brainrecovery-project.org/parents/brain-surgeries-to-stop-seizures/amygdalohippocampectomy/)

Spencer D, Burchiel K. Selective amygdalohippocampectomy. Epilepsy Res Treat. 2012; 2012:382095

# Section VII

## Pain Management Strategies

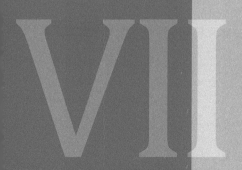

# 17 Spinal Cord Stimulator

*Ryan F. Amidon, Christ Ordookhanian, and Paul E. Kaloostian*

## 17.1 Symptoms and Signs

- Chronic back, leg, or arm pain (failed back syndrome or postlaminectomy syndrome)
- Sciatica
- Reduction of mobility from pain
- Pain and discomfort derived from consistent nerve irritation

## 17.2 Surgical Pathology

- Spine benign/malignant trauma
- Spine benign/malignant disorder
- Vascular benign/malignant lesion

## 17.3 Diagnostic Modalities

- Patient history
- Physical examination
- Neurologic examination
- MRI of spine
- CT of spine
- X-ray of spine
- PET of spine

## 17.4 Differential Diagnosis

- Cord compression
- Arachnoiditis
- Multiple sclerosis
- Spinal cord injury
- Failed back surgery syndrome
- Complex regional pain syndrome
- Stump pain
- Angina
- Peripheral vascular disease

## 17.5 Treatment Options

- Acute pain control with medications and pain management
- Physical therapy and rehabilitation
- If asymptomatic or mildly symptomatic with cord compression:
  - Surgical decompression and fusion of implicated segments if deemed suitable candidate for surgery
    - If poor surgical candidate with poor life expectancy, medical management recommended
- If asymptomatic without cord compression and no relief from other therapies:
  - Baclofen pump (permanent pump implant that delivers baclofen to spinal fluid, treating spasticity refractory to oral medications and chronic pain associated with moderate to severe spasticity)
    - Baclofen is a $GABA_B$ Receptor agonist, promoting muscle relaxation
    - Morphine may be used instead of baclofen
  - Spinal cord stimulation (masks nociception before it reaches the brain, resulting in non perception of pain)
    - Pain relief varies from person to person
    - Includes: (1) pulse generator with battery, (2) lead wire with 8 to 32 electrodes, and (3) remote control to adjust settings and turn the device on or off
    - Need a trial showing 50% pain relief with psychological clearance and no untreated drug addiction noted

## 17.6 Indications for Surgical Intervention

- No sufficient improvement of pain after nonoperative measures (physical therapy, medications/injections, pain management)
- Chronic pain after one or more spinal surgeries
- No perceived benefit from additional surgery, or risks too high
- No untreated depression or drug addiction
- A successful spinal cord stimulation trial was conducted
- Significant reduction in everyday activities due to symptoms

## 17.7 Surgical Procedure for Spinal Cord Stimulation

1. Informed consent signed, preoperative labs normal, no Aspirin/Plavix/ Coumadin/NSAIDs/Celebrex/Naprosyn/other anticoagulants and anti-inflammatory drugs for at least 2 weeks

2. Appropriate intubation and sedation and lines (if necessary) as per the anesthetist
3. Patient placed prone in neutral alignment on Jackson Table with all pressure points padded
4. Neuromonitoring not necessary
5. Time out is performed with agreement from everyone in the room for correct patient and correct surgery with consent signed
6. Prep areas of back and buttock where the leads and generator will be placed
7. Insert the electrode leads under fluoroscopic guidance (see ▶ Fig. 17.1)
    a. Make a small incision down the midline of back, exposing bony vertebra
    b. Perform laminotomy:
        i. Remove portion of bony arch, making room to place the leads
    c. Position leads/paddle in epidural space above spinal cord at specific level based on trial and confirmed on X-ray or fluoroscopy and secured with sutures
8. Run test stimulation if necessary
    a. Awaken the patient and test how well stimulation covers his or her pain areas
9. Once lead electrodes are in place, pass wire under the skin from the spine to the buttock, where generator will be implanted
10. Place pulse generator
    a. Make a small incision below the waistline
    b. Create a pocket for the generator beneath the skin
    c. Attach the lead wire to the pulse generator and position it within the skin pocket
11. Close the incisions with sutures and skin glue, applying a dressing

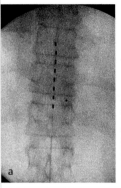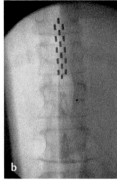

**Fig. 17.1** A trial electrode was inserted percutaneously into the T10–T12 midline to cover postsurgical radiculopathy (a). An insulated paddle electrode was then placed at T11–T12 (b) as they were determined to be the most effective location during the trial period. (Source: Surgical procedure. In: Sekhar L, Fessler R, eds. Atlas of Neurosurgical Techniques: Brain, Vol. 2. 2nd ed. Thieme; 2015).

## 17.8 Pitfalls

- Unpleasant tingling sensations
- Failure to sufficiently reduce pain
- Bleeding
- Infarction
- Blood clot formation
- Epidural hemorrhage, hematoma, infection, cord compression, and/or paralysis
- Battery failure and/or leakage
- Cerebrospinal fluid (CSF) leakage
- Seroma at implant site (may require drain)
- Lead migration
- Allergic response to implant materials
- Generator migration and/or local skin erosion
- Weakness, clumsiness, numbness, or pain below level of implantation

## 17.9 Prognosis

- Hospitalization rates depend on the type of procedure performed, preoperative examination status, and patient's age/comorbidities (same-day or following morning discharge is typical)
- Physical therapy and occupational therapy will be needed postoperatively, immediately and as outpatient to regain strength
- Do not bend, lift, or twist back or reach overhead for next 6 weeks
- Do not lift anything heavier than 5 pounds
- Abstain from strenuous activity
- Do not drive until follow-up appointment
- Do not drink alcohol
- Programming of pulse generator can be adjusted in follow-up appointment as needed

## Bibliography

Spinal cord stimulation. Mayfield Brain & Spine. (https://mayfieldclinic.com/pe-stim.htm)

# 18 Baclofen Pump/Morphine Pump

*Ryan F. Amidon, Christ Ordookhanian, and Paul E. Kaloostian*

## 18.1 Symptoms and Signs

- Chronic back, leg, or arm pain (failed back syndrome or postlaminectomy syndrome)
- Sciatica
- Reduction of mobility from pain
- Pain and discomfort derived from consistent nerve irritation
- Stiffened muscles
- Spasms

## 18.2 Surgical Pathology

- Spine benign/malignant trauma
- Spine benign/malignant disorder
- Vascular benign/malignant lesion

## 18.3 Diagnostic Modalities

- Patient history
- Physical examination
- Neurologic examination
- MRI of spine
- CT of spine
- X-ray of spine
- PET of spine

## 18.4 Differential Diagnosis

- Muscle spasticity
- Cord compression
- Arachnoiditis
- Multiple sclerosis
- Spinal cord injury
- Failed back surgery syndrome
- Complex regional pain syndrome
- Stump pain

- Angina
- Peripheral vascular disease
- Stroke

## 18.5 Treatment Options

- Acute pain control with medications and pain management
- Physical therapy and rehabilitation
- If asymptomatic or mildly symptomatic with cord compression:
  - Surgical decompression and fusion of implicated segments if deemed suitable candidate for surgery
    - If poor surgical candidate with poor life expectancy, medical management recommended
- If asymptomatic without cord compression and no relief from other therapies:
  - Baclofen pump (permanent pump implant that delivers baclofen to spinal fluid, treating spasticity refractory to oral medications and chronic pain associated with moderate to severe spasticity) (see ▶ Fig. 18.1)
    - Baclofen is a $GABA_B$ Receptor agonist, promoting muscle relaxation
    - Morphine may be used instead of baclofen
  - Spinal cord stimulation (masks nociception before it reaches the brain, resulting in non perception of pain)
    - Pain relief varies from person to person
    - Includes: (1) pulse generator with battery, (2) lead wire with 8 to 32 electrodes, and (3) remote control to adjust settings and turn the device on or off
    - Must perform a trial placement showing over 50% pain relief with psychological clearance and no untreated drug addiction or habituation

## 18.6 Indications for Surgical Intervention

- No sufficient improvement of pain after nonoperative measures (physical therapy, medications/injections, pain management)
- Chronic pain after one or more spinal surgeries
- No perceived benefit from additional surgery, or risks too high
- No untreated depression or drug addiction
- A successful injection trial was conducted, where baclofen or morphine was injected into spinal canal with a small needle
- Significant reduction in everyday activities due to symptoms

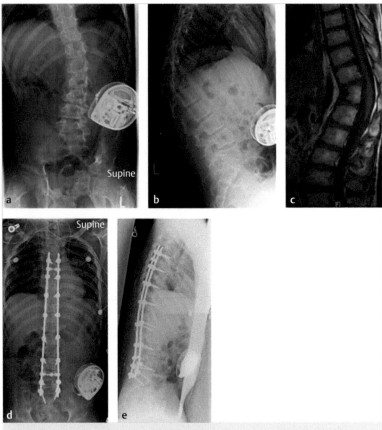

**Fig. 18.1** (a–e) A baclofen pump is visible in the radiographs of this teenage boy suffering from cerebral palsy and kyphosis. (Source: Surgical treatment. In: Heary R, Albert T, eds. Spinal Deformities: The Essentials. 2nd ed. Thieme; 2014).

## 18.7 Surgical Procedure for Intrathecal Baclofen Pump Insertion

1. Informed consent signed, preoperative labs normal, no Aspirin/Plavix/Coumadin/NSAIDs/Celebrex/Naprosyn/other anticoagulants and anti-inflammatory drugs for at least 2 weeks
2. Appropriate intubation and sedation and lines (if necessary) as per the anesthetist

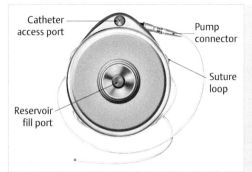

**Fig. 18.2** Illustration of baclofen pump demonstrating its different parts and their functions. (Source: Overview. In: Harbaugh R, Shaffrey C, Couldwell W, et al, eds. Neurosurgery Knowledge Update: A Comprehensive Review. 1st ed. Thieme; 2015).

3. Patient placed in lateral decubitus position in neutral alignment on Jackson Table with all pressure points padded
4. Neuromonitoring not necessary
5. Time out is performed with agreement from everyone in the room for correct patient and correct surgery with consent signed
6. Small stab incision made midline over spinous process of lumbar spine at L4–L5 region
   a. Lumbar puncture needed insertion into CSF-containing cavity and the catheter is advanced through the needle followed by immediate needle retraction
   b. Catheter is tunneled toward anterior incision in abdomen
7. Insert the pump:
   a. Perform incision over lower abdominal muscles
   b. Use self-retaining retractors to maintain sufficient accessible space
   c. Insert pump under covering of lower abdominal muscles using minimal dissection (see ▶ Fig. 18.2)
8. Fill the pump:
   a. Insert small catheter through a needle into spinal fluid space, and thread it upward
   b. Tunnel the catheter under the skin to abdomen, connecting it to the pump
   c. Fill the pump with baclofen or morphine and program it via computer to continuously release a predetermined dose
   d. Close the incision with sutures or surgical staples

# 18.8 Pitfalls

- CSF leakage
- Pain, numbness, weakness, or paralysis due to nerve damage

- Bleeding/injury to blood vessels
- Postoperative infection
- Meningitis
- Paralysis
- Catheter fracture or migration
- Pump malfunction

## 18.9 Prognosis

- Hospitalization rates depend on the type of procedure performed, preoperative examination status, and patient's age/comorbidities
  - Discharge possible after vital signs stabilize and patient returns to baseline functions
- Pump will need to be refilled every couple of months (1–6 months), depending on pump size, concentration, and dose. Its battery lasts 5 to 7 years.

## Bibliography

Baclofen Pump. University of Rochester Medical Center. (https://www.urmc.rochester.edu/neurosurgery/for-patients/treatments/baclofen-pump.aspx)

Penn RD, Savoy SM, Corcos D, et al. Intrathecal baclofen for severe spinal spasticity. N Engl J Med. 1989; 320(23):1517–1521

VIII

# 19 Ventriculoperitoneal Shunt

*Ryan F. Amidon, Christ Ordookhanian, and Paul E. Kaloostian*

## 19.1 Symptoms and Signs

- Gait disturbance
- Difficulty maintaining balance and walking
- Mild dementia
- Impaired bladder control
- Headache
- Fatigue
- Nausea
- Irritability
- Confusion
- Large head size
- Seizures
- Impaired vision
- Abnormal sleeping behavior
- Memory loss

## 19.2 Surgical Pathology

- Cranial benign/malignant trauma
- Cranial benign/malignant infection
- Cranial benign/malignant tumor
- Cranial benign/malignant surgical complication

## 19.3 Diagnostic Modalities

- Patient history
- Physical examination
- Neurological examination
- CT of brain (detect enlarged ventricles)
- MRI of brain (detect enlarged ventricles)
- Ultrasound of brain
- Cerebrospinal fluid (CSF) testing (predict shunt responsiveness, determine shunt pressure)
  - Lumbar or spinal tap
  - External lumbar drainage
  - Measure CSF outflow resistance

# 19.4 Differential Diagnosis

- Communicating hydrocephalus: CSF can still flow between ventricles, but gets blocked after exiting
  - Resulting from subarachnoid hemorrhage, head trauma, infection, tumor, or surgical complication
  - Normal pressure hydrocephalus (NPH)
  - Pseudotumor cerebri
- Noncommunicating hydrocephalus (obstructive hydrocephalus): CSF flow blocked along passage(s) connecting ventricles
- Congenital hydrocephalus vs. acquired hydrocephalus
- Hydrocephalus ex-vacuo: Occurs when stroke, degenerative diseases, or head trauma damages brain (brain tissue shrinkage may occur)

# 19.5 Treatment Options

## 19.5.1 Surgery if Deemed Suitable Candidate

- Determine overall prognosis and Karnofsky performance score
- If poor surgical candidate with poor life expectancy, medical management recommended
- Endoscopic third ventriculostomy (neuroendoscope visualizes ventricular surface and a hole is created in floor of third ventricle, allowing CSF to bypass obstruction and flow toward sites of resorption)
- Shunting (relieving fluid buildup responsible for hydrocephalus)
  - Types:
    - Ventriculoperitoneal (VP): Ventricular inflow, peritoneal cavity (abdomen) outflow
    - Lumboperitoneal (LP): Lumbar spine inflow, peritoneal cavity (abdomen) outflow
    - Ventriculopleural (VPL): Ventricular inflow, pleural cavity (lung) outflow
    - Ventriculoatrial (VA): Ventricular inflow, right atrium of heart outflow
  - Components:
    - Inflow/Proximal catheter (drains CSF from ventricles or subarachnoid space)
    - Valve mechanism (regulates differential pressure or controls flow through shunt tubing, connected to proximal catheter)
    - Outflow/Distal catheter (directs CSF from valve to abdominal or peritoneal cavity, heart, or other drainage site)

# 19.6 Indications for Surgical Intervention

- Gait disturbance
- Trauma or hemorrhage
- Normal pressure hydrocephalus
- Pseudotumor cerebri
- Ventricle size disproportionately larger than CSF in subarachnoid space
- Removal of spinal fluid through lumbar puncture or catheter results in temporary relief
- Intracranial pressure (ICP) or spinal fluid pressure monitoring demonstrates abnormal range or pattern of spinal fluid pressure or sufficiently elevated CSF outflow resistance

# 19.7 Surgical Procedure for Ventriculoperitoneal (VP) Shunt

1. Informed consent signed, preoperative labs normal, patient ceases intaking of NSAIDs (Naprosyn, Advil, Nuprin, Motrin, Aleve) and blood thinners (Coumadin, Plavix, Aspirin) 1 week prior to treatment
2. Appropriate intubation and sedation and lines (if necessary) as per the anesthetist
3. Place patient in supine position on operating table, head turned 90 degrees to contralateral side, and all pressure points padded
4. Neuromonitoring not needed
5. Time out is performed with agreement from everyone in the room for correct patient and correct surgery with consent signed
6. A urinary catheter may be placed to drain urine from bladder
7. Shave head (if necessary) where head incision will be performed
8. Perform incision(s) behind ear (two or three may be necessary):
   a. Drill occipital or frontal burr hole in skull
   b. Dissect through meninges, creating small opening
   c. Insert inflow/proximal catheter and move it to predetermined ventricle
   d. Insert outflow/distal catheter subcutaneously, tunneling it down to chest and ultimately peritoneal cavity (abdomen), using an endoscope
      i. Additional small cuts may be necessary to facilitate movement of catheter
   e. Insert shunt valve behind ear
9. Connect proximal and distal catheters to shunt valve behind ear
10. Close incisions with sutures or surgical staples and apply sterile bandage(s)

# 19.8 Pitfalls

- Postoperative infection
- Meningitis
- Subdural hematoma
- Blockage/Obstruction complications
- Shunt under-drainage complications:
  - Elevated ICP
  - Recurrence of hydrocephalus
- Shunt over-drainage complications:
  - Proximal shunt obstruction: Tissue sucked into holes of proximal catheter, reducing inflow
  - Headache/dizziness
  - Slit ventricle syndrome: Absence of CSF within ventricles combined with growing brain (potentially fatal ICP before ventricles can expand)
  - Subdural collections: Fluid accumulations between arachnoid and dura
  - Extradural collections: Fluid accumulations between dura and skull
  - Secondary craniosynostosis: Cranial defect where bony sutures of infant close too early
  - Cyst formation around shunt (see ▶ Fig. 19.1)
  - Double compartment syndrome (rare; see ▶ Fig. 19.2)

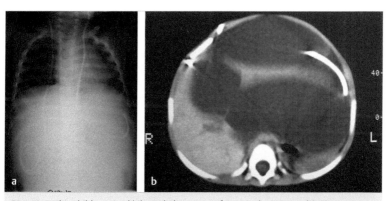

**Fig. 19.1** This child received bilateral placement of ventriculoperitoneal (VP) shunts (**a**). Months later, a cyst formed around the tips of both shunts as verified by CT (**b**). (Source: Rahalkar M. Complications of cerebrospinal fluid diversion (shunt) catheters: a pictorial essay. IJNS 2018;7(1):58–076).

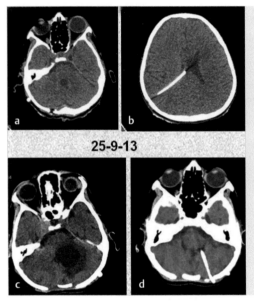

**Fig. 19.2** A teenage boy received ventriculoperitoneal (VP) shunts to treat hydrocephalus (**a, b**) after a choroid plexus papilloma operation. Within 7 months, double compartment syndrome developed (**c, d**) and the fourth ventricle was also shunted. (Source: Rahalkar M. Complications of cerebrospinal fluid diversion (shunt) catheters: a pictorial essay. IJNS 2018;7(1):58–76).

## 19.9 Prognosis

- Patient placed in post-anesthesia care unit (PACU) and ultimately hospitalized. Hospitalization rates depend on the type of procedure performed, preoperative examination status, and patient's age/comorbidities (typically 2–7 days)
- Physical therapy, occupational therapy, and other rehabilitation therapies recommended
- Pain management
- Headache, nausea, or vomiting, if present following the procedure, will warrant relevant medications

## Bibliography

Hydrocephalus. Johns Hopkins Medicine. (https://www.hopkinsmedicine.org/health/conditions-and-diseases/hydrocephalus)

Procedure S. Johns Hopkins Medicine. (https://www.hopkinsmedicine.org/neurology_neurosurgery/centers_clinics/cerebral-fluid/procedures/shunts.html)

Surgery: What to Expect—Implanting a Ventriculoperitoneal (VP) Shunt. Medtronic. (https://www.medtronic.com/us-en/patients/treatments-therapies/hydrocephalus-shunt/getting-a-device/surgery.html)

Systems S. Hydrocephalus Association. (https://www.hydroassoc.org/shunt-systems/)

Ventriculoperitoneal AY. (VP) Shunt Surgery. Memorial Sloan Kettering Cancer Center. (https://www.mskcc.org/cancer-care/patient-education/about-your-ventriculoperitoneal-vp-shunt-surgery)

Ventriculoperitoneal Shunting. MedlinePlus. (https://medlineplus.gov/ency/article/003019.htm)

# 20 Lumboperitoneal Shunt

*Ryan F. Amidon, Christ Ordookhanian, and Paul E. Kaloostian*

## 20.1 Symptoms and Signs

- Gait disturbance
- Difficulty maintaining balance and walking
- Mild dementia
- Impaired bladder control
- Headache
- Fatigue
- Nausea
- Irritability
- Confusion
- Large head size
- Seizures
- Impaired vision
- Abnormal sleeping behavior
- Memory loss

## 20.2 Surgical Pathology

- Cranial benign/malignant trauma
- Cranial benign/malignant infection
- Cranial benign/malignant tumor
- Cranial benign/malignant surgical complication

## 20.3 Diagnostic Modalities

- Patient history
- Physical examination
- Neurological examination
- CT of brain (detect enlarged ventricles)
- MRI of brain (detect enlarged ventricles)
- Ultrasound of brain
- Cerebrospinal fluid (CSF) testing (predict shunt responsiveness, determine shunt pressure)
  - Lumbar or spinal tap
  - External lumbar drainage
  - Measure CSF outflow resistance

# 20.4 Differential Diagnosis

- Communicating hydrocephalus: CSF can still flow between ventricles, but gets blocked after exiting
  - Resulting from subarachnoid hemorrhage, head trauma, infection, tumor, or surgical complication
  - Normal pressure hydrocephalus (NPH)
  - Pseudotumor cerebri (idiopathic intracranial hypertension)
- Noncommunicating hydrocephalus (obstructive hydrocephalus): CSF flow blocked along passage(s) connecting ventricles
- Congenital hydrocephalus vs. acquired hydrocephalus
- Hydrocephalus ex-vacuo: Occurs when stroke, degenerative diseases, or head trauma damages brain (brain tissue shrinkage may occur)

# 20.5 Treatment Options

## 20.5.1 Surgery if Deemed Suitable Candidate

- Determine overall prognosis and Karnofsky performance score
- If poor surgical candidate with poor life expectancy, medical management recommended
- Endoscopic third ventriculostomy (neuroendoscope visualizes ventricular surface and a hole is created in floor of third ventricle, allowing CSF to bypass obstruction and flow toward sites of resorption)
- Shunting (relieving fluid buildup responsible for hydrocephalus)
  - Types:
    ○ Ventriculoperitoneal (VP): Ventricular inflow, peritoneal cavity (abdomen) outflow
    ○ Lumboperitoneal (LP): Lumbar spine inflow, peritoneal cavity (abdomen) outflow
    ○ Ventriculopleural (VPL): Ventricular inflow, pleural cavity (lung) outflow
    ○ Ventriculoatrial (VA): Ventricular inflow, right atrium of heart outflow
  - Components:
    ○ Inflow/proximal catheter (drains CSF from ventricles or subarachnoid space)
    ○ Valve mechanism (regulates differential pressure or controls flow through shunt tubing, connected to proximal catheter)
    ○ Outflow/distal catheter (directs CSF from valve to abdominal or peritoneal cavity, heart, or other drainage site)

# 20.6 Indications for Surgical Intervention

- Gait disturbance
- Trauma or hemorrhage noted
- Ventricle size disproportionately larger than CSF in subarachnoid space
- Pseudotumor cerebri
- Removal of spinal fluid through lumbar puncture or catheter results in temporary relief
- Intracranial pressure (ICP) or spinal fluid pressure monitoring demonstrates abnormal range or pattern of spinal fluid pressure or sufficiently elevated CSF outflow resistance

# 20.7 Surgical Procedure for Lumboperitoneal (LP) Shunt

1. Informed consent signed, preoperative labs normal, patient ceases intaking of NSAIDs (Naprosyn, Advil, Nuprin, Motrin, Aleve) and blood thinners (Coumadin, Plavix, Aspirin) 1 week prior to treatment
2. Appropriate intubation and sedation and lines (if necessary) as per the anesthetist
3. Place patient in lateral decubitus position with arms raised above shoulders (avoiding localized compression) on operating table, and all pressure points padded
4. Neuromonitoring not needed
5. Time out is performed with agreement from everyone in the room for correct patient and correct surgery with consent signed
6. A urinary catheter may be placed to drain urine from bladder
7. Landmarks of interest:
   a. Iliac crest: L4–L5 cord level
   b. If epidural hemorrhage due to needle puncture, use L5–S1 level instead
8. Prep skin of lumbar area, flank, and abdomen
9. Perform longitudinal incision in midline
10. Carry dissection down to muscle fascia layer
11. Insert a Tuohy needle into thecal sac
    a. Needle bevel aligned in rostral–caudal direction
    b. Measure pressure if necessary
12. Insert catheter through Tuohy needle and into thecal sac for about 6–8 cm, allowing for some displacement upon needle removal
    a. Never withdraw catheter through needle once it has passed the tip to avoid shearing off the end of catheter
    b. If additional attempts are necessary, remove needle with catheter

13. Simultaneously access peritoneal cavity through laparoscopic or open approach, using flank incision
    a. A direct approach to peritoneum requires a more medial ventral incision
    b. Dissect through Scarpa fascia, innominate fascia, muscle layers, and transversalis fascia, until peritoneal membrane is reached
14. Valve placement (see ▶ Fig. 20.1):
    a. Perform flank incision and connect it to lumbar using catheter-tunneling instrument

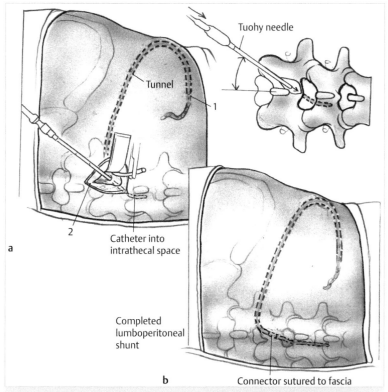

**Fig. 20.1** Illustrative guide to lumboperitoneal (LP) shunt placement: Lumbar, flank, and abdominal incisions are performed. (**a**) Demonstrates catheter insertion into the lumbar incision (labeled 2) to drain cerebrospinal fluid (CSF) from intrathecal space (abdominal incision is labeled 1). (**b**) Demonstrates insertion of valves and reservoirs at the midpoint of the tunneled catheter. (Source: Lumboperitoneal shunt for coccidiomycosis meningitis. In: Nader R, Berta S, Gragnanielllo C, et al, eds. Neurosurgery Tricks of the Trade: Spine and Peripheral Nerves. 1st ed. Thieme; 2014).

b. Bring spinal catheter to flank exposure, ensuring that it is not dislodged from thecal sac

c. Suture anchoring device to lumbar fascia to prevent displacement, with additional tubing as strain relief

d. Connect valve to the cut end of spinal catheter

e. Place additional tubing in similar fashion from the flank incision to abdominal incision

15. Ascertain flow from distal end of system before placement into peritoneal cavity

16. Apply purse-string suture in peritoneum around catheter to reduce displacement

17. Close incisions with sutures or surgical staples and apply sterile bandage(s)

## 20.8 Pitfalls

- Postoperative infection
- Subdural hematoma
- Meningitis
- Blockage/Obstruction complications
- Shunt under-drainage complications:
  - Elevated ICP
  - Recurrence of hydrocephalus
- Shunt over-drainage complications:
  - Proximal shunt obstruction: Tissue sucked into holes of proximal catheter, reducing inflow
  - Headache/Dizziness
  - Slit ventricle syndrome: Absence of CSF within ventricles combined with growing brain (potentially fatal ICP before ventricles can expand)
  - Subdural collections: Fluid accumulations between arachnoid and dura
  - Extradural collections: Fluid accumulations between dura and skull
  - Secondary craniosynostosis: Cranial defect where bony sutures of infant close too early

## 20.9 Prognosis

- Patient placed in postanesthesia care unit (PACU) and ultimately hospitalized. Hospitalization rates depend on the type of procedure performed, preoperative examination status, and patient's age/comorbidities.

- Physical therapy, occupational therapy, and other rehabilitation therapies recommended
- Pain management
- Headache, nausea, or vomiting, if present following the procedure, will warrant relevant medications

# Bibliography

Hydrocephalus. Johns Hopkins Medicine. (https://www.hopkinsmedicine.org/health/conditions-and-diseases/hydrocephalus)

Lumboperitoneal Shunt Placement Technique. Medscape. (https://emedicine.medscape.com/article/1890515-technique)

Shunt Procedure. Johns Hopkins Medicine. (https://www.hopkinsmedicine.org/neurology_neurosurgery/centers_clinics/cerebral-fluid/procedures/shunts.html)

Shunt Systems. Hydrocephalus Association. (https://www.hydroassoc.org/shunt-systems/)

# 21 Ventriculopleural Shunt

*Ryan F. Amidon, Christ Ordookhanian, and Paul E. Kaloostian*

## 21.1 Symptoms and Signs

- Gait disturbance
- Difficulty maintaining balance and walking
- Mild dementia
- Impaired bladder control
- Headache
- Fatigue
- Nausea
- Irritability
- Confusion
- Large head size
- Seizures
- Impaired vision
- Abnormal sleeping behavior
- Memory loss

## 21.2 Surgical Pathology

- Cranial benign/malignant trauma
- Cranial benign/malignant infection
- Cranial benign/malignant tumor
- Cranial benign/malignant surgical complication

## 21.3 Diagnostic Modalities

- Patient history
- Physical examination
- Neurological examination
- CT of brain (detect enlarged ventricles)
- MRI of brain (detect enlarged ventricles)
- Ultrasound of brain
- Cerebrospinal fluid (CSF) testing (predict shunt responsiveness, determine shunt pressure)
  - Lumbar or spinal tap
  - External lumbar drainage
  - Measure CSF outflow resistance

# 21.4 Differential Diagnosis

- Communicating hydrocephalus: CSF can still flow between ventricles, but gets blocked after exiting
  - Resulting from subarachnoid hemorrhage, head trauma, infection, tumor, or surgical complication
  - Normal pressure hydrocephalus (NPH)
- Noncommunicating hydrocephalus (obstructive hydrocephalus): CSF flow blocked along passage(s) connecting ventricles
- Congenital hydrocephalus vs. acquired hydrocephalus
- Hydrocephalus ex-vacuo: Occurs when stroke, degenerative diseases, or head trauma damages brain (brain tissue shrinkage may occur)

# 21.5 Treatment Options

## 21.5.1 Surgery if Deemed Suitable Candidate

- Determine overall prognosis and Karnofsky performance score
- If poor surgical candidate with poor life expectancy, medical management recommended
- Endoscopic third ventriculostomy (neuroendoscope visualizes ventricular surface and a hole is created in floor of third ventricle, allowing CSF to bypass obstruction and flow toward sites of resorption)
- Shunting (relieving fluid buildup responsible for hydrocephalus)
  - Types:
    - Ventriculoperitoneal (VP): Ventricular inflow, peritoneal cavity (abdomen) outflow
    - Lumboperitoneal (LP): Lumbar spine inflow, peritoneal cavity (abdomen) outflow
    - Ventriculopleural (VPL): Ventricular inflow, pleural cavity (lung) outflow
    - Ventriculoatrial (VA): Ventricular inflow, right atrium of heart outflow
  - Components:
    - Inflow/Proximal catheter (drains CSF from ventricles or subarachnoid space)
    - Valve mechanism (regulates differential pressure or controls flow through shunt tubing, connected to proximal catheter)
    - Outflow/Distal catheter (directs CSF from valve to abdominal or peritoneal cavity, heart, or other drainage site)

# 21.6 Indications for Surgical Intervention

- Gait disturbance NPH
- Known cause with tumor or trauma

- Ventricle size disproportionately larger than CSF in subarachnoid space
- Removal of spinal fluid through lumbar puncture or catheter results in temporary relief
- Intracranial pressure (ICP) or spinal fluid pressure monitoring demonstrates abnormal range or pattern of spinal fluid pressure or sufficiently elevated CSF outflow resistance
- Multiple failures of ventriculoperitoneal (VP) shunts
- Peritoneum not acceptable site for distal catheter placement
- Failure of ventriculoatrial (VA) shunts

# 21.7 Surgical Procedure for Ventriculopleural (VLP) Shunt

1. Informed consent signed, preoperative labs normal, patient ceases intaking of NSAIDs (Naprosyn, Advil, Nuprin, Motrin, Aleve) and blood thinners (Coumadin, Plavix, Aspirin) 1 week prior to treatment
2. Appropriate intubation and sedation and lines (if necessary) as per the anesthetist
3. Place patient in supine position in neutral alignment on operating table with all pressure points padded
4. Neuromonitoring not needed
5. Time out is performed with agreement from everyone in the room for correct patient and correct surgery with consent signed
6. A urinary catheter may be placed to drain urine from bladder
7. Proximal catheter may be placed frontally or through occipital burr hole:
   a. If frontally, place hemostat or temporary suture to prevent CSF egress
8. Place positive end-expiratory pressure valve in anesthesia circuit to maintain lung inflation during pleural catheter placement, avoiding pneumothorax
9. Perform skin incision at third or fourth rib off the midline (in the same line used for passage of distal catheter) and insert self-retaining retractors
10. Dissect toward pleura through muscles of anterior chest wall and intercostal muscles
11. Connect shunt entirely before opening the pleura (see ▶ Fig. 21.1):
    a. Connect proximal catheter to shunting device
    b. Ascertain flow of CSF from distal catheter
    c. Make pleural egress with long hemostat and place about 20 cm of tubing into pleural space, under direct vision
12. Irrigate wound and close incisions with sutures or surgical staples, applying sterile bandages

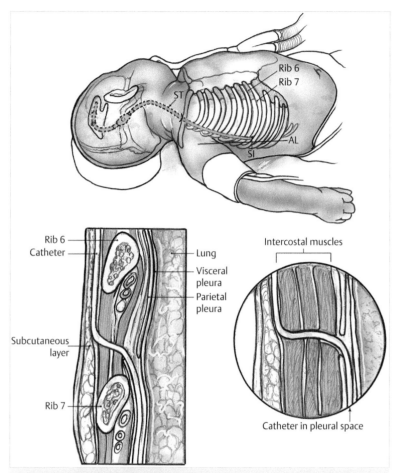

**Fig. 21.1** Illustration of ventriculopleural (VPL) shunt positioning in child. (Source: Ventriculopleural shunts. In: Nader R, Gragnaniello C, Berta S, et al, eds. Neurosurgery Tricks of the Trade: Cranial. 1st ed. Thieme; 2013).

## 21.8 Pitfalls

- Postoperative infection
- Meningitis
- Pleural effusion

- Subdural hematoma
- Pulmonary complications
- Blockage/Obstruction complications
- Shunt under-drainage complications:
  - Elevated ICP
  - Recurrence of hydrocephalus
- Shunt over-drainage complications:
  - Proximal shunt obstruction: Tissue sucked into holes of proximal catheter, reducing inflow
  - Headache/Dizziness
  - Slit ventricle syndrome: Absence of CSF within ventricles combined with growing brain (potentially fatal ICP before ventricles can expand)
  - Subdural collections: Fluid accumulations between arachnoid and dura
  - Extradural collections: Fluid accumulations between dura and skull
  - Secondary craniosynostosis: Cranial defect where bony sutures of infant close too early

# 21.9 Prognosis

- Patient placed in post-anesthesia care unit (PACU) and ultimately in the intensive care unit (ICU). Hospitalization rates depend on the type of procedure performed, preoperative examination status, and patient's age/comorbidities
- Physical therapy, occupational therapy, and other rehabilitation therapies recommended
- Pain management
- Headache, nausea, or vomiting, if present following the procedure, will warrant relevant medications

# Bibliography

Hydrocephalus. Johns Hopkins Medicine. (https://www.hopkinsmedicine.org/health/conditions-and-diseases/hydrocephalus)

Küpeli E, Yilmaz C, Akçay S. Pleural effusion following ventriculopleural shunt: case reports and review of the literature. Ann Thorac Med. 2010; 5(3):166–170

Shunt Systems. Hydrocephalus Association. (https://www.hydroassoc.org/shunt-systems/)

Shunt Procedure. Johns Hopkins Medicine. (https://www.hopkinsmedicine.org/neurology_neurosurgery/centers_clinics/cerebral-fluid/procedures/shunts.html)

# 22 Ventriculoatrial Shunt

*Ryan F. Amidon, Christ Ordookhanian, and Paul E. Kaloostian*

## 22.1 Symptoms and Signs

- Gait disturbance
- Difficulty maintaining balance and walking
- Mild dementia
- Impaired bladder control
- Headache
- Fatigue
- Nausea
- Irritability
- Confusion
- Large head size
- Seizures
- Impaired vision
- Abnormal sleeping behavior
- Memory loss

## 22.2 Surgical Pathology

- Cranial benign/malignant trauma
- Cranial benign/malignant infection
- Cranial benign/malignant tumor
- Cranial benign/malignant surgical complication

## 22.3 Diagnostic Modalities

- Patient history
- Physical examination
- Neurological examination
- CT of brain (detect enlarged ventricles)
- MRI of brain (detect enlarged ventricles)
- Ultrasound of brain
- Cerebrospinal fluid (CSF) testing (predict shunt responsiveness, determine shunt pressure)
  - Lumbar or spinal tap
  - External lumbar drainage
  - Measure CSF outflow resistance

## 22.4 Differential Diagnosis

- Communicating hydrocephalus: CSF can still flow between ventricles, but gets blocked after exiting
  - Resulting from subarachnoid hemorrhage, head trauma, infection, tumor, or surgical complication
  - Normal pressure hydrocephalus (NPH)
- Noncommunicating hydrocephalus (obstructive hydrocephalus): CSF flow blocked along passage(s) connecting ventricles
- Congenital hydrocephalus vs. acquired hydrocephalus
- Hydrocephalus ex-vacuo: Occurs when stroke, degenerative diseases, or head trauma damages brain (brain tissue shrinkage may occur)

## 22.5 Treatment Options

### 22.5.1 Surgery if Deemed Suitable Candidate

- Determine overall prognosis and Karnofsky performance score
- If poor surgical candidate with poor life expectancy, medical management recommended
- Endoscopic third ventriculostomy (neuroendoscope visualizes ventricular surface and a hole is created in floor of third ventricle, allowing CSF to bypass obstruction and flow toward sites of resorption)
- Shunting (relieving fluid buildup responsible for hydrocephalus)
  - Types:
    - Ventriculoperitoneal (VP): Ventricular inflow, peritoneal cavity (abdomen) outflow
    - Lumboperitoneal (LP): Lumbar spine inflow, peritoneal cavity (abdomen) outflow
    - Ventriculopleural (VPL): Ventricular inflow, pleural cavity (lung) outflow
    - Ventriculoatrial (VA): Ventricular inflow, right atrium of heart outflow
  - Components:
    - Inflow/proximal catheter (drains CSF from ventricles or subarachnoid space)
    - Valve mechanism (regulates differential pressure or controls flow through shunt tubing, connected to proximal catheter)
    - Outflow/distal catheter (directs CSF from valve to abdominal or peritoneal cavity, heart, or other drainage site)

## 22.6 Indications for Surgical Intervention

- Gait disturbance
- Known cause for hydrocephalus (i.e., trauma or hemorrhage)
- Ventricle size disproportionately larger than CSF in subarachnoid space
- Removal of spinal fluid through lumbar puncture or catheter results in temporary relief
- Intracranial pressure (ICP) or spinal fluid pressure monitoring demonstrates abnormal range or pattern of spinal fluid pressure or sufficiently elevated CSF outflow resistance
- Multiple failures of ventriculoperitoneal (VP) shunts
- Peritoneum not acceptable site for distal catheter placement

## 22.7 Surgical Procedure for Ventriculoatrial (VA) Shunt

1. Informed consent signed, preoperative labs normal, patient ceases intaking of NSAIDs (Naprosyn, Advil, Nuprin, Motrin, Aleve) and blood thinners (Coumadin, Plavix, Aspirin) 1 week prior to treatment
2. Appropriate intubation and sedation and lines (if necessary) as per the anesthetist
3. Place patient in supine position on operating table, all pressure points padded
   a. Positioning influenced by location of proposed shunt placement or existing shunt system (the most favorable site for ventricular catheter placement will determine patient's position)
   b. Bolster shoulders to facilitate subcutaneous passage of shunt catheter and access to prospective feeding vein
   c. Be prepared to access a second vein if initial vessel proves difficult (i.e., ipsilateral subclavicular region in addition to neck)
4. Neuromonitoring is not needed
5. Time out is performed with agreement from everyone in the room for correct patient and correct surgery with consent signed
6. A urinary catheter may be placed to drain urine from bladder
7. If proximal catheter placed frontally:
   a. A portion of distal shunt tubing secured to outflow port of unidirectional shunt valve
   b. Perform 1 cm vertical retroauricular incision and pull tubing subcutaneously out through this incision
   c. Place hemostat or temporary suture to prevent CSF egress

8. If proximal catheter is placed through occipital burr hole:
   a. Tunnel distal shunt tubing directly to proposed site of entry for vascular access
9. Access appropriate vessel for atrial catheter positioning using percutaneous (Seldinger technique) or open vascular cutdown technique
   a. Ultrasonographic guidance may be used
   b. Internal jugular vein (IJV) is the most common access vessel:
      i. Puncture skin one to three fingerbreadths above clavicle, between heads of sternocleidomastoid muscle, using 20 or 22 gauge needle
   c. If subclavian vein access is chosen:
      i. Entry site inferior to clavicle, at junction of middle and lateral third of the bone
10. After cannulation of the vessel:
    a. Pass flexible guide wire through the needle
    b. Position the tip in the superior vena cava (SVC) or cardiac atrium, under fluoroscopic guidance
    c. Guide wire positioned within heart indicated by instability on electrocardiography (ECG)
11. Remove needle
12. Perform a nick incision to facilitate dilator entry
    a. Load peelaway sheath on the dilator and pass them together into the vessel
    b. Occasional advancing and retracting of guide wire ensures dilator is following wire's subcutaneous course
13. Remove dilator and guide wire
14. Pass shunt tubing down peelaway sheath
15. Pass distal shunt well beyond the lower atrium before splitting and removing the peelaway sheath
16. Pull back catheter to appropriate final position, flush with heparinized saline, and connect to proximal shunt system (see ▶ Fig. 22.1)
17. Open approach can also be used:
    a. Perform cutdown to IJV, applying purse-string suture on anterior wall of vein
    b. Perform stab incision inside purse-string
    c. Place catheter directly into vein
    d. Tie suture down around catheter to prevent back-bleeding
18. Alternatively, the transverse facial vein may be isolated as it enters the IJV:
    a. Divide transverse facial vein
    b. Pass shunt down into IJV
    c. Secure catheter to transverse facial vein using a tie, preventing back-bleeding
19. Verify location of distal catheter tip using fluoroscopy

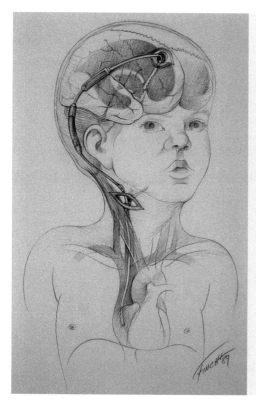

**Fig. 22.1** Illustration of ventriculoatrial (VA) shunt positioning in child. (Source: Operative procedure. In: Goodrich J, ed. Pediatric Neurosurgery. 2nd ed. Thieme; 2008).

a. Position tip of distal catheter in middle to lower atrium, at about T6 vertebral body level
b. If tip is insufficiently visualized, inject small volume of radiopaque contrast material
20. Trim proximal and distal catheters
21. Verify flow of CSF through proximal catheter system
22. Flush distal catheter with heparinized saline
23. Connect distal catheter to proximal catheter using a straight connector
24. Irrigate incisions with antibiotic-impregnated saline
25. Close incision in layers, using sutures or surgical staples and apply sterile bandage(s)

## 22.8 Pitfalls

- Postoperative infection
- Subdural hematoma

- Meningitis
- Immune-complex glomerulonephritis
- Pulmonary hypertension
- Endocarditis
- Delayed intracranial hemorrhage
- SVC thrombosis
- Intramuscular migration of venous catheter
- Blockage/Obstruction complications
- Shunt underdrainage complications:
  – Elevated ICP
  – Recurrence of hydrocephalus
- Shunt overdrainage complications:
  – Proximal shunt obstruction: Tissue sucked into holes of proximal catheter, reducing inflow
  – Headache/Dizziness
  – Slit ventricle syndrome: Absence of CSF within ventricles combined with growing brain (potentially fatal ICP before ventricles can expand)
  – Subdural collections: Fluid accumulations between arachnoid and dura
  – Extradural collections: Fluid accumulations between dura and skull
  – Secondary craniosynostosis: Cranial defect where bony sutures of infant close too early

## 22.9 Prognosis

- Patient placed in post-anesthesia care unit (PACU) and ultimately hospitalized. Hospitalization rates depend on the type of procedure performed, preoperative examination status, and patient's age/comorbidities.
- Physical therapy, occupational therapy, and other rehabilitation therapies recommended
- Pain management
- Headache, nausea, or vomiting, if present following the procedure, will warrant relevant medications

## Bibliography

Hankinson T, Miller J. Ventriculoatrial Shunt Placement Technique. Medscape. 2018. (https://emedicine.medscape.com/article/1895753-technique)

Hydrocephalus. Johns Hopkins Medicine. (https://www.hopkinsmedicine.org/health/conditions-and-diseases/hydrocephalus)

Shunt Procedure. Johns Hopkins Medicine. (https://www.hopkinsmedicine.org/neurology_neurosurgery/centers_clinics/cerebral-fluid/procedures/shunts.html)

Shunt Systems. Hydrocephalus Association. (https://www.hydroassoc.org/shunt-systems/)

# Index

Note: Page numbers set in **bold** or *italic* indicate headings or figures, respectively.

**313**

# T

Tarlov cyst **145**, **146**, 147,
**148**, **149**
- diagnostic modalities for
145, 146, 147
- differential diagnosis of
145
- excision of 148
- pitfalls in procedures for
149
- prognosis of 149
- surgical indications for
148
- surgical pathology of
145
- surgical procedure for
posterior sacral spine
148
- symptoms and signs of
145
- treatment options for
146
Third ventriculostomy,
endoscopic 291, 297,
303, 308
Thoracic corpectomy and
fusion 41, **42**, 43, **44**,
**45**, **46**, **47**, **48**, **62**, **63**,
**64**, **65**, 66, 67, **68**, **69**,
**70**, 82
- corpectomy approaches
in 43, 44, 45, 46, 47, 65,
68, 69
-- anterior (thoracoscopic)
43
-- posterior (transpedicular) 43, 44, 47, 69
-- posterolateral (lateral
extracavitary) 43, 46, 68
-- retropleural (anterolateral) 43, 44, 45, 65
- for capillary hemangi-
oma 82
- for myelopathy 67
- in elective procedures
62, 63, 64, 65, 69, 70
-- diagnostic modalities in
63
-- differential diagnosis in
63
-- indications for 65
-- pitfalls in 69
-- prognosis in 70

-- surgical pathology in 63
-- surgical procedures for
65
-- symptoms and signs for
62
-- treatment options in 64
- in trauma 42, 44, 48
-- diagnostic modalities in
42
-- differential diagnosis in
42
-- indications for 44
-- pitfalls in 48
-- prognosis in 48
-- surgical pathology in 42
-- symptoms and signs for
42
-- treatment options in 42
Thoracic decompression and
fusion **37**, **38**, **39**, 40,
**41**, **48**, **49**, 50, 51, 52,
53, **55**, **56**, **57**, **58**, **59**,
**62**, **70**, **71**, **72**, 73, 74,
**75**, **77**, **78**, **79**, 312
- corpectomy with 312
- in elective procedures
57, 58, 59, 62
-- diagnostic modalities in
57
-- differential diagnosis in
57
-- indications for 59
-- pitfalls in 62
-- procedure for posterior
spine 59
-- prognosis in 62
-- surgical pathology in 57
-- symptoms and signs for
57
-- treatment options in 58
- in trauma 37, 38, 39, 40,
41
-- diagnostic modalities in
37
-- differential diagnosis in
37
-- indications for 38
-- pitfalls in 41
-- prognosis in 41
-- surgical pathology in 37
-- surgical procedure for
posterior spine 39
-- symptoms and signs for
37
-- treatment options in 38

- transsternal approaches
for 48, 49, 51, 55, 56,
70, 71, 72, 73, 77, 78, 79
-- anterior 51, 55, 73, 77
-- diagnostic modalities in
49, 71
-- differential diagnosis in
49, 71
-- indications for 51, 73
-- in elective procedures
70
-- in trauma 48
-- pitfalls in 56, 78
-- prognosis in 56, 79
-- surgical pathology in 49,
71
-- symptoms and signs for
48, 70
-- treatment options in 49,
72
- transthoracic approaches
for 40, 48, 49, 50, 51,
52, 53, 56, 70, 71, 72,
73, 74, 75, 78, 79
-- anterior 50, 51, 72, 75
-- anterolateral 52
-- diagnostic modalities in
49, 71
-- differential diagnosis in
49, 71
-- indications for 51, 73
-- in elective procedures
70
-- in trauma 48
-- lateral 53
-- pitfalls in 56, 78
-- prognosis in 56, 79
-- surgical pathology in 49,
71
-- symptoms and signs for
48, 70
-- treatment options in 49,
72
Thoracic outlet decompression 61
Thoracic spine **37**, **38**, **42**,
**44**, **48**, **49**, 50, **51**, **57**,
60, **79**, 312
- elective procedures for
57
- multilevel pathology of
60
- surgical approaches to
50

retroperitoneal transpsoas approach for 162